HOSPICE

HOSPICE

CREATING NEW MODELS OF CARE
FOR THE TERMINALLY ILL

Parker Rossman

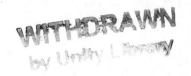
FAWCETT COLUMBINE • NEW YORK

To Jean
without whom...

Foreword

> Behind it followed in an endless string
> A train so long, I scarce could deem it true
> Death had undone such hosts past numbering.
>
> DANTE

Death is a seemingly insufferable scandal to modern man. It testifies against his Promethean illusions, hovers invisibly but insistently over his work and merriment and insinuates itself into the plasticized ambience he has fabricated to keep it out.

Pascal wrote, "Since men could not do away with death they decided not to think about it." Everywhere the walls of denial have gone up. We worship youth and health; we exact medicine's magical powers to defeat death; we immerse ourselves in works, sense, sensations, and spectacles. When we do exhibit death openly in the press, movies and novels, we do not confront, rather we so flaunt it in its violent forms, that we only anesthesize and shock, nauseate. By fantasticizing death we deny it once again.

The physician and nurse can less easily ignore death, who is their constant enemy and partner. Yet in their special way, they deny it too. The incurable patient is quietly set aside, no longer talked to, visited infrequently and condescendingly, and declared "beyond" the help of medicine.

Families and friends must erect special defenses when someone they love forces the reality of death into their midst. We are embarrassed when someone we love forces on our consciousness the realization that life, as Dante said, is "a racing unto death." So we consign them to the pre-mausoleum of the hospital. Meanwhile we protest that there they can receive the "best care", excusing ourselves from too close a participation in the scandal of dying.

Yet, as Troisfontaines wrote in *I Do Not Die,* "death spies on men every day and has its foot at the door." When the verdict of cancer or any undeniably incurable illness is pronounced, our hiding place is suddenly revealed. The foot at the door is inside the house! Death is no longer a deniable abstraction or an obscenity which afflicts others. We ourselves become the bearers of the scandal from which even friends and family recoil.

Even more horrendously, with the intuition of incurability, the act of dying is immediately thrust upon us. Unlike death itself, which must remain a mystery, the act of dying is visible. And ineluctable. It must be experienced, whatever may be our opinion of the mystery of death itself. The lifelong personal and social cult of denial is poor preparation, indeed, for this awesome confrontation.

Yet somehow, the act of dying too must be assimilated and made a part of the life that remains if the afflicted person is not to become an object. The act of dying must be both *human* and *humane.* To be *human* it must be understood, consciously assimilated and given a personal quality and shape by the dying person himself. To be *humane,* all who assist, aid and collaborate in the act must provide what is necessary to make the last act a truly human one—to relieve pain, listen, provide those things which have meaning for the dying person, and permit him or her to make the major decisions on how, when and under what conditions to die.

Can the act of dying be made both human and humane in the contemporary world where so many things militate against it? This is the question which the Hospice movement described in this book answers confidently and competently, with an unequivocal yes! It does so despite the many things which now contravene that answer: the continuing denial by professionals, patients, and friends, the subtle isolation from ordinary human affairs, the efforts to "protect" the patient against the fact of his dying. The whole apparatus of modern hospital care seems designed to create a nonperson of the "terminal" patient and to sequester him as a slightly indecent failure of modern technology. The only way he can serve is discreetly and efficiently to pass out of his life, relieving everyone of the embarrassment of his dying.

The Hospice movement vigorously stands against this aseptic walling off of the dying human from himself and other humans. Instead it offers a carefully designed regimen of "loving care" based in an environment sensitively attuned to recognizing the needs and even the "rights" of the dying. It addresses those needs and rights with a caring regimen of pain relief, personal and family counselling, attractive surroundings and sees to all those things which will put the patient in charge of his own dying as much as possible. Home care and hospitalization in a special unit are dovetailed to reenforce the aim of making the act of dying human and humane, and even, a creative one.

The author describes the origins, development, operation, and problems of the New Haven-Branford Hospice, the first to be established in this country outside the religious institutions dedicated to the care of incurable patients. He shows how the Hospice derived its major ideas from the St. Christophers and St. Josephs Hospices in England and how those programs have been modified. The history of care of the terminally ill is reviewed, the needs and rights of the dying patient are clearly spelled out, together with the program of care followed both at St. Christophers and at New Haven.

The book should be an essential reference for the audience to which it is addressed: those communities and individuals interested in establishing special units for the care of dying cancer patients. Everything is covered—the origins of the movement, the varieties of programs and institutional settings, the roles of physicians, nurses, social workers, psychiatrist and chaplain as individuals and team members, and the legal and fiscal problems yet to be settled. The book is an indispensable vademecum for anyone contemplating establishing a hospice.

While this book has its special utility for those who care for the dying cancer patient, its message of concerned "loving" care is equally significant for other forms of medical care—especially of the chronically ill. All patients share, to some degree, the same needs and rights so urgently underscored for the cancer patient. Perhaps the greatest contribution of this book will be to show again how drastically we must alter medical education and the organization of medical care to encompass the principles of humane and human care for all patients.

The challenges for medical, nursing and health profession educators are direct, specific, and inescapable as they are for administrators, boards of trustees and public policy makers. The ideal of patient-oriented, patient-centered, and patient-directed medical care is, perhaps, the most difficult unmet challenge before us today. In showing how the failure to attend to these dimensions frustrates, depersonalizes and dehumanizes the care of the dying patient, the hospice movement alerts all of us to a signal deficiency which no amount of elaborate technology, systems organization, or managerial efficiency can obliterate. Only persons can care, and without caring even the hospice idea becomes just another formula.

In the end, it is the loving concern, dedication, and unswerving determination of all who have carried through the New Haven-Branford Hospice that illuminates this book. I hope that spirit will inspire other communities to establish their own versions of the Hospice idea and to incorporate those same principles in the everyday care of all patients.

EDMUND D. PELLEGRINO, M.D.
President, Yale-New Haven Medical Center
Professor of Medicine, Yale University

Acknowledgments

Special appreciation and credit for assistance in preparing this book should be given to more people than can be listed here, but particularly I may mention my creative editor, Robert Roy Wright; along with Miriam Gillitt, research assistant to Dr. Balfour Mount of the Palliative Care Service at Royal Victoria Hospital; Yeates Conwell, Jr., medical student; Dr. Raymond Duff of Yale University Medical School; Dr. Melvin J. Krant, director of the Medical Center cancer programs at the University of Massachusetts Medical School in Worcester; Dr. Josefina B. Magno of the Vincent T. Lombardi Cancer Research Center in Washington; Connecticut legislator Irving Stolberg; Prof. Jay Katz of Yale Law School; Mrs. Florence Wald, former dean of Yale Nursing School; Dr. David Duncombe, chaplain of Yale Medical School; Ruth Knollmueller for information on Visiting Nurse Associations and her nursing experience; and for much help from the following members of the hospice program at St. Luke's Hospital in New York: Clinical Specialist Roberta Paige, Dr. Philip E. Gordon, Chaplains David Pyle and Carleton Sweetser. Although proper appreciation cannot begin to be given to enough persons related to the New Haven Hospice, my special thanks are due to Frank Kryza II, who brought great vision and intellectual gifts to his position as director of Public Relations, and to Dr. Morris Wessel, Chaplain Edward Dobihal, Mrs. Sally Bailey (whose insight into the problems of the dying was helpful to me even before she came to the hospice program), Natalie Tyler, Department of Research and Evaluation, especially for bibliographical help, and lastly to hospice pharmacy consultant Dr. Arthur G. Lipman of Yale-New Haven Hospital and the University of Connecticut School of Pharmacy.

Dr. Cicely Saunders and others are responsible for corrections to bring up to date the paperback edition.

—PARKER ROSSMAN

Niantic, Conn.
December, 1978

Contents

Introduction

People do not fear death so much as they fear dying, a process which for many persons—young as well as old—is a slow, painful, and very lonely experience. Dying persons often have weeks or even months to live after it is determined that cure is impossible. This should be a time of sustaining relationships with family and friends so that a meaningful life can be enjoyed to the end. Instead, despite all the technological advances in health care—or as Constance Holden puts it, despite "the millions of dollars this country is pouring into the war against cancer—little heed is paid to the plight of the victims once their individual battles are lost." For example, she says, of the 700,000 people diagnosed as having cancer each year, two out of three die of the malignancy. Thus terminally-ill persons often find themselves feeling isolated, miserable, helpless, and out of control of their life. For, "despite the growing concern about death and dying in this country, there is not much understanding of the needs of dying people." [1]*

Indeed, in many cases the medical profession's zeal to prolong life has merely succeeded in prolonging death in a cold-blooded, impersonal way. Instead of a person's life coming to a human, dignified, and meaningful climax, it ebbs away in a

---

* Superior figures refer to Chapter Notes at end of text.

hospital isolation ward, hooked into machines, with jabbing needles instead of loving touch. At worst, such treatment can be cruel and inhuman punishment; at best, it is an environment designed for science, and not for human life. As places of cure, hospitals must perhaps be designed with scientific efficiency for the convenience of nurses and physicians, not for patients. Almost anyone is willing to surrender some freedom in order to be cured of a serious disease, and to save one's life if one can become free and happy again. But when they are terminally ill and ready to die, most people want to be in a happier environment.

The hospice concept, as pioneered in England; in Montreal, Canada; in New Haven, Connecticut, and elsewhere, offers a model which suggests there are ways to reduce the pain and misery of dying persons and their families, demonstrating how a caring environment can be created for the terminally ill. These terminally ill are by no means only elderly persons— indeed, half of them are under age 50, with many being children. Speaking out of her experience at St. Christopher's Hospice in England, Dr. Cicely Saunders [2] talks of death as the last frontier—where physical, mental, and spiritual needs come together. She and her hospice colleagues have a point of view which can be helpful not only to health-care professionals but to all persons, especially as we contemplate our own death or face a decision about the care of a dying person in our own family.

There is a vast new literature on death and dying which examines taboos and attitudes—held by physicians and nurses as well as by the public—which have helped to create the misery that many dying persons now experience in hospitals. Dr. Elisabeth Kübler-Ross [3] pioneered in listening to dying persons themselves in order to obtain their thoughts and suggestions so as to help physicians, clergy, families, and other involved persons to understand the experiences of the terminally ill, their needs—and their wish for a more human and dignified environment for their last days. Our culture has sought to pretend that death does not happen or at least that is is something morbid which one should never think about. Each of us hopes to slip off into a sweet death while sleeping or to have the happy sort of death my father had. In his latter years my father had built up his physical strength and health with outdoor work and hiking. In his retirement he had a series of interesting short-term jobs which helped him to feel young. One position took him from Oklahoma to the Colorado mountains he loved so well, another to live in New England near his grandchildren for a time. He and Mother also wanted to visit their other grandchildren, who were in Japan, so they booked space on a tramp steamer which stopped for a day or two in nearly every free port on the east coast of Asia. Dad returned with insights and photographic slides which opened a new career of travel talks which he greatly enjoyed. Then, one day in the second decade of his retirement, Dad telephoned his chess crony to say: "Last night you beat me, but I'm coming over to checkmate you tonight." Dad was feeling buoyant because he had completed his share of fund raising for his college graduation class and he wanted to celebrate the fact that everyone he had solicited had made a contribution. His chess friend was not feeling well and really didn't want to play that evening, but Dad was full of enthusiasm. So that evening they played a fine game of chess, and Dad dropped dead, instantly, triumphantly, when he won. No pain, no lingering suffering, just a fine, dignified climax to an enjoyable life. As much as the family misses him, we cannot but be grateful for that.

Most people save and plan for old age with the hope and expectation of a good life until they die, but the medical profession, with the best intentions, seems at many points to have lost sight of this goal of a "good life" in its efforts to prolong life at any cost. As press debates have recently reminded us, the result has frequently been a prolonging of death and thus making dying more tedious, difficult, and miserable. Many persons who would have died earlier have prolonged periods of terminal misery precisely because excellent medical care is available to more and more people—indeed, if society is willing to spend millions of dollars on each person, a great many lives could be extended indefinitely by hooking the individuals' heart and lungs to machines. But what kind of life would this be to go on for months or years with the patient perhaps unconscious or wishing to be so!

There is another kind of subtle misery which is far less controversial. As Dr. Richard Lamerton [4] has pointed out, there is a tendency for physicians and nurses to become more and more neglectful of a patient once he or she has been labeled incurable. The physician who is trained to cure, and who is committed to preventing death, may simply leave the dying person in the hands of nurses, once he feels there is nothing more he can do, with the result that the patient sometimes feels abandoned. And young nurses—particularly those who have had little experience with dying patients—may also find such persons to be a problem and an embarrassment. Often even family members withdraw, with less frequent visits, uncertain what to do other than leave the terminally-ill person alone in a "dark and haunted corner of dreams and drug imagery" which is real suffering.

Edward Dobihal, Chaplain of Yale-New Haven Hospital and a member of the Yale Divinity School faculty; Florence Wald, former dean of the Yale School of Nursing, along with several others, were profoundly influenced by the thought of Dr. Kübler-Ross and the work of Dr. Saunders and her associates in England, because their observation of the suffering of dying persons had made clear the need for a *demonstration model* which might facilitate what Chaplain Dobihal called the "prophetic task" [5] of providing a better environment for the terminally ill. At different times both Dobihal and Mrs. Wald went to England to study the hospice movement. After they had returned to New Haven they joined forces with others in an experiment—the creation of an institution to serve the terminally ill which could serve as a center for teaching, for staff training, and for spreading the hospice concept and point of view in America. Federal funding was secured to underwrite the experimental program in New Haven. In 1977 this program is still in a provisional stage, but it has advanced to the point that persons from across the continent are visiting New Haven to study this American adaptation of the British hospice movement. Indeed, people from England have also visited New Haven to study American experience and adaptations which are reported in this volume. In the fall of 1975 a first consultation was held in New Haven for persons from thirty or more American communities which were launching similar or alternative experiments aimed at providing a better and more dignified life for terminally-ill persons.

This book is addressed primarily to those persons concerned with establishing hospice-type institutions or programs in their communities, but also it is for the general public—who sometime will die—as well as for families of the terminally ill. It also will be of great interest to clergy, social workers, health professionals, and other community leaders responsible for the planning and funding of social services.

The hospice program must be founded upon excellence in medical care, a type of medical science chiefly characterized by the sophisticated management of severe pain and other debilitating symptoms. Beyond that, however, the concern is also essentially pastoral, reflecting as it does the same sort of concern that in the past has led many religious persons to found hospitals and nursing orders. Chaplain Dobihal speaks of the hospice as being a "model to stimulate new forms of care for, and ministry to, persons who have chronic degenerative disease and a limited life span." He uses such terminology because of his faith and focus on helping people live, not die. He points out that despite all the excellent books and lectures on death and dying, there is still a great resistance and taboo in our society which causes persons to turn their eyes aside from the terminally ill, and which causes society often to shunt off the dying into a corner where they can be ignored. As people contemplate death, many of them fear that isolation and pain, they worry that unnecessary and uncomfortable treatments will be continued after being no longer necessary, thus diminishing the quality of life and family associations in their last days. They have only to visit the wards of almost any hospital to see people taped down, plugged into machines, isolated from grandchildren and pets, lonely and in miserable circumstances. The real fear of death for many persons therefore is a dread of this loss of control over their life, of not even being consulted when crucial decisions are made between alternatives of treatment and care.

One physician said: "The basic aim in this hospital is to get people cured and out of the hospital as soon as possible. We are not running a luxury hotel devoted to making patients happy, but we are organized for efficiency to mobilize all possible resources for cure." The dying person who lingers in such a hospital is seen by the medical staff as one of their failures. And scientists do not wish to fail—even when there is no further chance of sustaining a meaningful and happy life the tempo of efficiency is maintained or even increased with more discomfort, pain, machines, more needles stuck in veins, more impossible expense—and all for nothing in so many cases. As the clergy and psychiatrists seek to relieve anxieties, they are being increasingly frustrated as to how to help families that are caught up in the misery of such prolonged deaths.

The hospice, by contrast, provides an interdisciplinary model which focuses first upon expert palliative medical treatment, not for cure but to care for the person and the family and to allow them to participate in the care and in the decisions about alternatives. "The hospice," Dobihal says, "is not merely another institution. Our first effort is to keep dying persons with their family as much as possible. Our primary task is *to listen to them*, to discover with them what their needs are. But whether patient are at home or in a facility, the emphasis is upon freeing the family to be together, rather than their being wearied with burdens beyond their strength." [6] The hospice provides a way for health care personnel, clergy, and others, to work together as a team to help the dying and their families. Patients and family members are also seen to be members of the team. Families can help and can teach other families, and patients can help and teach other patients, what they are learning about living and dying.

Dobihal points out that the Branford Hospice in New Haven, as is true of hospice-type programs described here, is not to be seen as an institution which can be copied in other communities. "We have no blueprints to share that would be just right in another place, but visitors here *can* discover a point of view —that the dying can be made comfortable by palliative treatment in many instances, and that they can be loved in a way that can enrich the end of their life. Other communities will design 'caring environments' in a style unique to their own needs and situation." [7] In the New Haven area, careful study showed that there were enough terminally ill people to justify a hospice facility, where in another area the program might well be limited to home care, or to a wing of an existing hospital as back-up for a home care program.

Many of the social services of society are justified on the grounds that they restore persons to productive work. Dying persons, by contrast, are valued not merely because their families value them, Dobihal says, but because they are seen as children of God and therefore important to all. "The hospice program is a real demonstration of love and a proclamation of the religious message that death as well as life has meaning. We help people live their lives out fully and richly and thus preach by example that human life is valued whether or not it has productive use for society." The hospice program values and affirms families and strengthens family ties to the end of life. Terminally-ill people sometimes live for many months; during this time they can establish close relationships with children and grandchildren if an enabling and loving climate is provided to replace the environment of taboo and withdrawal which leads so many to be embarrassed, not knowing what to say or do in the presence of the dying. *Newsweek* Magazine told the story of one hospice patient who had refused to go off to an impersonal institution to die among strangers. Instead—enabled to be free of pain—he stayed at home to share the end of his life with his wife and children. He was even able to say: "I'm enjoying life again." [8] C. S. Lewis described a similar experience with his dying wife: "It is incredible the happiness . . . we had together after all hope was gone. How long, how tranquilly, how nourishingly, we talked together that last night." [9] Such an experience does not mean that all difficulties and suffering are gone when pain—physical, mental, social, and spiritual—is carefully tended to, but it does suggest that there are alternatives yet to be explored to make life more bearable and to give the dying more dignity. As Dobihal says: "The world will not be made perfect for those who are dying nor for those continuing to live. The hospice will not be a perfect environment, but we can give patients and families the best care that we can devise and then share our discoveries with those who are serving the dying elsewhere. At least the hospice can be—in the words of one of my dying friends at a hospice I visited in England—a place where people care and have time to share." [10]

1

Mrs. Morgan Wanted to Die at Home

What should be done with someone like Mrs. Alma Morgan, bedridden for two years and dying with inoperable cancer? [1] Blind, frightened, tearful, she and her family had to face months of waiting for death. Mrs. Morgan had literally worn herself out in taking care of a dying husband. After his death she had a few good years of strength, when she could live alone and care for herself despite her diabetes and failing eyesight. But when she was struck down with cancer *and* blindness, Emma, her widowed daughter, had to come to live with her and take care of her. Emma could adequately take care of her mother when her two boys were home from college, but at other times her mother was too heavy for her to turn alone. And when Mrs. Morgan needed to be taken to the dentist or to the hospital, Emma had to phone for an expensive ambulance or else obtain assistance from a home-care agency which never seemed able to respond promptly when she needed help.

Mrs. Morgan often wept because she didn't want to be such a burden on her daughter, who had to leave her own home and friends for a semi-isolated life with her mother, for Mrs. Morgan remembered her own misery at trying to cope with a dying husband without adequate counsel and help. On the other hand, in her blindness and fear, Mrs. Morgan was unwilling to let her daughter leave her bedside for even a few hours of rest and relaxation. She complained that an employed substitute, and even the visiting nurse, did not take care of her properly. Time after time she awakened her daughter in the middle of the night. She kept her running from morning to night until Emma finally collapsed under the burden. Emma's children came home from college to rescue their mother, and to make sure she got the rest and care she needed they called a family council meeting to decide what to do. Mrs. Morgan's sister was willing to help, but her husband would not permit her to stay in another town for long. Her brother, caught up in a divorce, could not leave his job, and it was little help for him to fly in on Saturday and back on Sunday.

Yet Emma had to have some rest and help, so Mrs. Morgan —screaming her protests—was taken to a nursing home. It was difficult there, at first, for the family to sort out her legitimate complaints from her agonizing desire to be at home. She wanted her dog. The nursing-home rules would not permit her to turn on her radio for the question-and-answer talk show which was her favorite late-night activity. She complained that she had no one to talk to, as she was sharing a room with a woman who spoke only Hungarian. Her doctor rarely came to see her. The nursing-home attendants didn't give her the right medicine at the right time. She complained that often no one would come when she desperately needed help. The family, seeing no alternative way of care for Mrs. Morgan, turned away from her complaints, feeling that these were in the same mode as her continual complaining at home—until one day she went into a coma because the staff failed to give her an insulin shot.

The family's rage, when they came to the nursing home, doctor in tow, was met with rage. The nursing-home staff said that Mrs. Morgan was so demanding, and required such continual and complicated care, that she could no longer stay. She must, they said, be taken to a hospital. Mrs. Morgan and her family had felt that they could not afford the nursing home, much less a $120-a-day hospital. And the physician said that the hospital was crowded, with priority given to people who could be cured. He helped the family negotiate with home-care agencies for more help for Emma. After much crying and weeping—with everyone mad at everyone else—the family agreed that Emma would employ some help to provide for her time off. Though a number of persons replied to the notice placed in the parish church paper asking for help, none stayed very long. Some were incompetent, some were undependable. The best woman employed—who did assume a great deal of the burden of physical work—herself became ill, and the next best one brought a burden of emotional problems of her own which she had to keep talking about, although it upset Mrs. Morgan and Emma, who had enough emotional problems of their own. Mrs. Morgan was increasingly in pain from her cancer, though her physician said the problem was largely in her mind, largely as a result of her unfortunate experience in the nursing home.

Even after enough help was available in the home, Emma collapsed again, partly because of the emotional burden of her mother's continual weeping and complaining. Desperately needing someone to talk to, Emma went to her mother's pastor, a newly-arrived priest in the huge parish, who came immediately to meet Mrs. Morgan, and to declare that he saw no alternative but for her to be taken to the hospital to die. Isn't that what hospitals are for? he asked. He telephoned Mrs. Morgan's doctor to argue about it. When Emma's sons came home for the week end, they agreed. In a crisis, they said, one turns to experts and the hospital is the place of expertise. In their fatigue from the situation and feeling incompetent, the family could only agree to do whatever the doctor would advise. When thus put on the spot to make a new decision, the physician saw that the family felt itself checkmated. It would be easier for him to see Mrs. Morgan from time to time if she was in the hospital, he said, so he made the decision, much to the relief of everyone—except Mrs. Morgan herself who begged to stay at home. He had her moved to the hospital "for tests." Mrs. Morgan was fully aware, and said so, that to get her into the hospital the doctor had to pretend that she was not terminally ill. She dreaded the hospital, partly because of the misery her husband had endured there. She said she was prepared to die at home with her souvenirs, her dog, her favorite phonograph records, and the memories that lingered around favorite possessions. Her tears were bitter when she was taken off in an ambulance against her will.

Many Mrs. Morgans

Less than a third of terminally-ill patients die at home, even fewer in major urban centers. Yet, as Mrs. Morgan expressed it so eloquently, the hospital is only a cage for the person whose life can no longer be extended in any meaningful way by hospitalization. When asked to express her feelings she told of a wild bird her older brother had caged when she had been a small child. She said that as a child she had thought it cruel to keep the wild bird in the cage, but had not really known why the bird sickened until she found, at the end of her life, how empty and meaningless everything was when she was "caged in the hospital." Society's growing awareness of the importance of environment—especially as bearing upon life quality—is increasingly manifest in concern for the climate of the classroom, the home, the workplace. For example, attention is increasingly given to the proper sort of environment for the growth and happiness of a preschool child. "The difference between home and hospital at the end of life," Mrs. Morgan said, "is the difference between life in a beautiful garden or underground in a coal mine." There is a sense in which she died psychologically in the ambulance on the way to the hospital, for she knew that she would never return to her home and life. She described her time in the hospital as a sort of purgatory, a time between life and death, "a time of empty waiting." As a free, responsible human being, why couldn't she have been given more choice in how to live the last part of her life?

One might argue on the basis of economics—the waste of Mrs. Morgan's money and of society's medical and financial resources—that it was foolish to move her into expensive hospital space against her will. But families are usually prepared to make every financial sacrifice, in the name of love, to secure the best possible care for loved ones. Indeed, Mrs. Morgan's neighbors were vocally critical of her family for delaying so long in moving her to the hospital. The neighbors said that when it came to proper care for dying persons there was no place for penny pinching. And the family finally refused to listen to Mrs. Morgan's own wishes precisely because they saw themselves as thinking too much about cost. Each member of the family, in his or her own way, felt guilty about the lack of time, energy, and skill, to take care of Mrs. Morgan. The easiest way to escape from guilt was finally to say: "Hang it! We'll get her the best care money can buy, regardless of the cost!" Also, by turning the problem over to someone else, each member of the family could relax. Mrs. Morgan's daughter could get a job again, and everyone could return to normal existence, free from the anxiety involved in trying to take care of her.

For all of the sensory deprivation suggested by Mrs. Morgan's thought that life in the hospital was like living underground in a coal mine or like a bird in a cage, the most important aspect of human environment is the quality of personal relationships. The question of *where* and *how* one dies is intertwined with the attitudes and behavior of each and all of the persons one experiences. Rather than generalizing about whether or not Mrs. Morgan could or should have remained to die at home, we will look in specific detail at the things said and done by people who surrounded her and took care of her, and what their alternatives might have been. Must so many Mrs. Morgans die in institutions when they would rather be at home?

What Dying People Think Is Crucial

People like Mrs. Morgan, dying in hospitals, complain that much of their misery is due to the fact that no one ever listens to them. Dr. Elisabeth Kübler-Ross therefore began to ask terminally-ill people about their problems, needs, feelings, worries, desires.[2] In several remarkable books, reporting on the experiences of the dying, she has provided information for physicians, clergy, families, nurses, and others, which is not only of common-sense value but also has provided an insightful foundation for further research into the attitudes and practices of professionals who deal with dying persons. She has opened the way to new alternatives for terminally-ill people, especially to make possible more meaningful lives to the end. One should not be surprised, therefore, to learn that she found human beings want to be loved as persons, rather than be treated as cases, as if the disease were more important than the person. Along with the magnificent advance of scientific medicine, something human seems to have been lost.

In an earlier time, Mrs. Morgan probably would have died at a younger age, perhaps of smallpox or pneumonia. Her family is grateful for the years which medical science added to her life, even if it did mean ending up in old age with her body riddled with cancer. Somehow, in its zeal to do everything, to work another miracle, the medical profession did not know how to give Mrs. Morgan the simple peace, companionship, comfort and freedom from pain which she wanted for her last days. This would not have been true in an earlier time when physicians took it for granted that there came a time when palliative care was all that was needed. Mrs. Morgan had her own long-thought-out plan for how she wanted to die. Her house was full of souvenirs. She had saved something from nearly every beautiful moment of her life—a napkin, for example, from the restaurant where her husband had asked her to marry him; a poorly mimeographed order of service from the church she had attended with her mother the Sunday before her mother had died; a marble she had begged from a boy she adored in the sixth grade. No one else knew what these bits and pieces of junk meant or why she had saved them, but it had been her plan throughout to save these souvenirs for the last hours of her life. The thought had first come to her when she was a teen-ager, of how nice it would be at the end of her life to touch all the mementos she had saved from her past, to aid her in reliving and summing up the joys of her life. So when she pleaded, as they took her to the hospital the last time, to stay home to die with her *things*, she could not even explain this in a way that her family considered important. Mrs. Morgan was ashamed—since they had often laughed about the way her house was littered with such trash—that she had spent her life building to a climax of remembering which was now being denied her!

Perception of Needs

Mrs. Morgan's family and physician may have shown too little perception and sensitivity to what she *wanted* because they felt they knew—better than she—what she *needed*. Her physician felt that she should be kept alive by artificial means, including being fed with a tube in her veins, when actually she was so ready to die that she wanted to stop eating. In the eyes of hospital staff she was a stubborn old woman who refused to eat, who never thanked them for services, and who instead always griped and complained that she wanted to go home, where she could hear small children playing in the yard next door. To live one day when those children would bring her flowers they picked in the yard meant more to her than extending her life a dozen lonely days in the hospital. But in defining her needs, no one else included her *need* for those dandelions. She knew quite well, for the most part better than anyone else, what she really needed, and her endless tears which so exasperated the hospital staff were not merely childish behavior at not getting what she wanted. The nurses told her that she was a spoiled, misbehaving old woman who caused them more trouble than any other patient on the floor. Because of her fear and anxiety, Mrs. Morgan needed loving, and not in the abstract. She needed to be touched and hugged, which was almost impossible the way she was rigged up in Intensive Care. She needed someone to listen when she was crying and saying mean things. She needed assurances that she was not abandoned, which, in turn, meant a physician who would come when she asked for him, a family which would discuss with her how things were being disposed of now that her house was being sold. She needed to talk about her fears, hopes, symptoms, and to be involved in the discussion of pros and cons with reference to her treatment and care. Even if the hospital staff had no means of doing nor any intent to do what she wanted, she needed to feel that she had been consulted.

The hospital staff, her physician, her family, and Mrs. Morgan could all agree on the words to describe her basic need: *a caring environment.* But they differed widely on what was meant by those words. To sensitive nurses and perhaps even to Emma, it meant TLC (tender loving care) of Mrs. Morgan's body. To Mrs. Morgan herself, although she thought it meant being in her own home, it actually meant sensitivity in her relationships, being with people who saw, in human terms, that life worth sustaining was more than a breathing lung and a beating heart. She needed to have her spiritual and emotional needs monitored by the hospital staff as carefully as they monitored her body fluids, temperature, and blood pressure. This, in turn, would have meant seeing the importance of making it possible for her to have more of her souvenirs and possessions with her at the hospital, if indeed she was to stay there until she died.

Mrs. Morgan fought with the only weapon she had, striving to make things as unpleasant as possible for those who took care of her. Although she was not a well-educated woman, she was well read. She had taken a great interest in student protest movements and pacifism. One day she confronted her physician with a question which he was unwilling to discuss—indeed, he found disturbing and shocking: "Isn't it *consciousness* that is the precious thing about human life, and not the spark of life which we readily kill in insects and animals we eat?" Mrs. Morgan was referring to the unconscious patient in the next bed, whose noises, treatment, machines, and even presence were more than she could endure, since it all reminded her of her husband's last days in the hospital. Her overwhelming need was to be moved elsewhere, to get away from the sounds and sights of a life that not only kept her tearful and fearful but also gave her nightmares. At this time she told the chaplain that her body was being well cared for, but that her consciousness was being abused.

Since her need, even in her own perception of it, was for a view and understanding of human life which she could feel was shared by her "captors," she no doubt would have been most appreciative of Houston Smith's suggestion that such a view requires "one to move from an understanding of life as survival or existence to see life as fulfillment." [3] Those who equate life with survival, he says, are restricted in their capacity to minister to the dying—for what meaning is possible in this perspective? Dr. Cicely Saunders sees at the heart of the hospice concept a change of attitude which is needed throughout the medical establishment: from negative to positive in regard to death and the possibility of a meaningful life to the hour of death. [4] In the natural order of things death does not need to be difficult for the very old and the very ill, she says, "for the body has a wisdom of its own, and dying can become a truly peaceful process." For this reason "there comes a time when tea is better than tubes," when life quality should take precedence over meaningless prolongation of bodily functioning. In fact, she suggests, happy patients live longer and hospital staffs are often aware of cases in which someone like Mrs. Morgan simply gives up and dies because life has become miserable and meaningless. In other words, the children next door with the dandelions might have been more effective in prolonging Mrs. Morgan's life than all the hospital equipment. For this reason, and not only in hospice programs, a new attention is now frequently being given to occupational therapy with dying persons: games, parties, films, children playing and so on. Dr. Saunders says, for example, that far from being a distraction to the terminally ill, children seem to feel a great affinity for tired and old persons and are frequently ready to bring affection and joy into their lives.

Rights of the Dying

In a century when society has paid much attention to human and civil rights, the helpless members of the community, such as the sick, the aged, and children, have not received a fair share of attention. Mrs. Morgan, for example, because she was blind and helpless, was treated by her family and physician almost as if she no longer had any rights at all. Since any of us may find ourselves in that situation, encouragement should be given to the development of a bill of rights for terminally-ill people.[3] Much of the ethical discussion about patients' rights is not helpful, for it is founded upon such theoretical arguments as, for example, "truth as an absolute value" in Kantian terms. And discussion of the "right to life" or a "right to die" tends to a legalism which leaves out compassion and love. Our focus, therefore, is not so much upon legal questions—important as they are—regarding the right to privacy or to access to the world outside the hospital, and so on. Rather we focus on the human needs of persons like Mrs. Morgan, not with a rigid view of rights but as human beings needing care and concern.

1. *The right to be heard.*

Some of Mrs. Morgan's bitterest tears in the hospital were the result of her strong feeling that no one, not even the family members she loved most, seemed to listen to her any more. She felt that they did not hear her when she spoke of things important to her. Such things as: where she wanted to die; how she wanted to spend her time and live until she died; the doctor didn't come to see her often enough; she thought the night nurse was cruelly impatient with her tears. She wanted to gripe and complain about little things, human things which seemed unimportant to them when they argued with her instead of listening. She needed the "hearing companionship" of people who thought that her feelings were important enough to be heard and understood. (To have someone willing to listen, even when one's thoughts seem to ramble incoherently or seem childish, is one way to feel that one's dignity as a person is being affirmed.) Mrs. Morgan's daughter, who spent a great deal of time at the hospital, always came prepared to tell her mother all the news and gossip about neighbors and community. Indeed, Emma spent a wearying amount of time on the phone before she came to the hospital, gathering information about things her mother had been interested in. Emma was therefore irritated that her mother seemed to prefer to ramble on about things Emma had heard a thousand times—such as what Mrs. Morgan had written on a napkin the night she had rightly guessed her future husband was going to propose. Emma felt that Mrs. Morgan was slipping into a world of past memories instead of keeping in touch with the present, real world of friends and neighbors. Emma told her children:

"Grandmother is getting this morbid feeling about death, always wanting to talk about the past." Emma herself was the one with attitudes toward death that made it impossible for her to face it with her mother in a warm, understanding way.

So Mrs. Morgan could not persuade her daughter, the one person close to her who knew many of the long-gone friends and family members, to join her in her reveries and remembrances. On the day Emma made the great effort involved in bringing a semi-invalid neighbor for a one-time-only visit to her mother, Mrs. Morgan, in the neighbor's presence, tried to force Emma to bring a "box of her junk," as Emma put it, to the hospital. Mrs. Morgan tried hard to get her daughter to listen to this authentic last request. Had Emma but listened, she would have found that her mother's tears dried up for the hour. Indeed, her mother would have laughed with Emma as she happily handled each of the souvenirs she had requested, as an aid to remembering the happy times which were almost forgotten. Emma listened, instead, to hospital authorities who took a very dim view of having a trunk brought from Mrs. Morgan's attic to the hospital.

2. *A second right of the dying person is to be told all the facts.*

This means more than just the truth about the patient's medical condition. In the midst of the current debate over whether all cancer patients should be told the truth if they are incurable, and discussion over the right of patient and family to see medical records, certain other aspects of truth-telling have been overlooked. For example, Mrs. Morgan's cancer physician carefully kept her informed at each stage of her diagnosis and treatment, as her family physician had earlier done with the diabetes. She was not, however, treated with equal candor by her family. As Mrs. Morgan's eyesight failed, her family let her slip more and more into ignorance about what was going on. The most crucial injustice, for Mrs. Morgan, was in the financial area. Over and over she asked for an accounting of her funds and property and was always told: "Never mind, Mama, we're taking care of everything." Emma and others in the family thought Mrs. Morgan would worry and would be terribly unhappy if she knew that she no longer had adequate financial resources to pay for all of her medical care. They tried, unsuccessfully, to fool her into thinking that she had more money than she had, and because they did not, and would not, talk with her frankly about such things they simply compounded her worry.

Emma frankly admitted after her mother's death that had Mrs. Morgan known the true facts about the burden of the hospital bills she would have used the money shortage as an excuse to demand to be taken home immediately. "We were sure," Emma said, "that mother would be more relaxed and happy in the hospital if we didn't bother her about financial matters." But Emma could not fool her mother about money any more than her physician could have fooled Mrs. Morgan about her cancer. Mrs. Morgan had been certain she had cancer even before the diagnosis was completed, and the official word that she had terminal cancer came actually as a relief from the tension which had resulted from uncertainty. No one, however, gave her that relief from the tension caused by her financial worries, or seemed to notice that she was tense and unhappy about this even to the day she died. Medically, in addition to the truth about one's condition, a patient often has the right to know more about alternative forms of treatment which may be under consideration.

3. *The terminally-ill person has the right to share in decision-making—including the right to refuse treatment.*[4]

Indeed, all mentally-competent persons have this right. At this time the courts have not yet made it clear that a person has a right earlier in life to sign a "Living Will" which would prevent being kept alive by artificial means.[5] The right of competent persons to refuse treatment, however, or to choose between alternative treatments is as basic as is the right to decide what to eat, how to spend one's time, and where to live. Society has given much thought to the question of who has the right to make decisions for helpless and incompetent persons, but there seems to be a reversal in modern times in the respect due to older persons and in the tender concern due to people who are dying. Mrs. Morgan was like most older persons today, and like many younger terminally-ill people, when she said that although her mind was sharp and her judgment was as good as it ever had been, her family had begun treating her as a child again in making the decision to move her to the hospital against her will. Mrs. Morgan herself had always been what she called a "fair person" who never made decisions for others without consulting them and taking into account their own wishes and feelings. She had always considered it important to consult her grown children on her major decisions, even after they had left home. With her strong sense of family solidarity, Mrs. Morgan might have gone to the hospital happily had all the alternatives been discussed openly with her, for, as much as she wanted to stay at home, she did not want to be selfish. But she felt that she had alternatives to propose, to the hospital and for caring for her at home, which were never even discussed.

Her physicians probably took too narrow a view of medical care, by assuming they were not to be consulted on family matters but only on alternative types of treatment: for example, whether to operate, to give medication of one kind or another, whether to use some new type of therapy. Because the physician recognizes the fallibility of his own judgment, he will generally consult with other doctors on such medical matters. And he will generally consult with the patient and family, saying, for example: "There is a 50-50 chance if I operate. Shall I do so?" In such cases the surgeon explains the alternatives to his patient, along with their consequences.

Otherwise he must play God by deciding upon his own responsibility how to treat the patient.

The vigilance which a patient and family must show in order to make sure they know and understand all the possible alternatives is illustrated by the ignorance of Mrs. Morgan and her family over pain-control measures in the hospital. Over and over again, Mrs. Morgan's physician told her and the family that he was doing all he could to control the agonizing pain caused by her cancer. But this was simply not true. Either he was not in fact aware of research on pain control and did not want to reveal his ignorance or else he was careless and prejudiced—in the sense of some of the nurses who had been taught that it was wrong to use heavy enough dosage of drugs as to possibly cause addiction, even in the hours of dying. Mrs. Morgan was not unconscious or senile. She was a brilliant and mentally-alert woman with good judgment. She could have understood a clear explanation of the procedures in pain control, including alternative possibilities and perils. Emma could have been given a medical article on pain control to read to her, so that the two of them could have actively cooperated with the nurses, and could have known what to do when one nurse was negligent.

4. *Dying persons have the right to share in their own care, to maintain control over their own life, and to have the quality of life which they choose.*

Mrs. Morgan was probably completely unaware of legal discussions over the "right to leave" a hospital, yet she once complained: "This hospital acts as if it is master and I am slave. I'm a captive here with no rights." In discussing a similar situation, Krant suggests that a person ultimately has two possibilities in the way he or she faces suffering and dying.[6] Either a patient like Mrs. Morgan finds a way to stay in reasonable control of her destiny or she allows herself to be caught up "in futility and hopelessness," giving herself over to the control of others. Mrs. Morgan was terribly unpopular with nurses, doctors, and others at the hospital because of her crying and raging, but none of them—not even her family—seemed to realize that she was acting as a child because against her will they were treating her as a child. In fact, however, even a child should be given more control over his or her life. As Bloom points out,[7] families tend to see a hospital as a custodial institution that takes over the management of a dying person so as to free the family from worry and care, and the family therefore frequently assents to a control over the patient that would never be tolerated at home. Bloom further notes that the extent to which a patient is able to keep some meaningful control over his or her life is greatly determined by the choice of hospital. In other words a terminally-ill person may be treated in widely different ways in one hospital as opposed to another, or even from ward to ward in the same hospital. Mrs. Morgan's family had been aware, in choosing a nursing home, that the quality of such institutions varies considerably, but they had no comparable opportunity or data to use in choosing a hospital. In truth they had little choice but to let the physician move Mrs. Morgan into the hospital which was most convenient for him. And in choosing nursing home and hospital the family evidently gave no thought to Mrs. Morgan's right to keep some control over her own life within the institution.

Mrs. Morgan was used to being asked: "Would you care for a cup of tea?" But in the hospital, she said, the tea was poured down her whether she wanted it or not: "It's time for your tea, so drink it now while I have time to help you." No one ever said: "Would you like to sit up now to rest your back?" She was always told, no matter how she felt: "You must sit up a while now." No one ever asked: "Is there anything you would like?" She was, she said, not supposed to like anything that wasn't on the official schedule or routine. No one on the ward seemed sensitive or informed as to what blind people can and want to do for themselves. But worse, she said, was the hospital staff's rigid emphasis on efficiency before all else, which—in a way she thought to be almost relentlessly cruel—continually reinforced her sense of lack of freedom to do anything or to decide anything for herself.

5. *Dying people have a right to die when their body and spirit are ready.*

Somewhere along the line—and all of society shares the blame—many members of the medical profession have become confused over the difference between neglectful failure to save life on one hand, and the unnecessary prolonging of dying on the other. The euthanasia issue underlies a discussion of patients' rights, since many people—if they take control of the aspects of their living which are related to dying—are likely to accept a sort of "passive euthanasia." Many people feel that to live well requires that the choice of death be available to them on their own terms. The hospice movement, without attempting to resolve euthanasia issues, seems to keep terminally-ill persons in the sort of situation which will make them want to live as long as they can. At the same time, it must be recognized that society can wreck itself by neglecting the rights of the young and the living and proceeding to spend too large a share of its financial resources on prolonging the lives of terminally-ill persons by artificial means. Never before in history has society had the capacity to extend for months and years the lives of so many people who will never again be conscious or have any life of quality or meaning. Should hundreds of thousands or even millions of dollars be spent to prolong the empty life of such persons? In this context some theologians and ethicists are asking hard questions about the meaning of life and death; some are suggesting that these persons each have their own unique perception of when they are going to die or ought to die, and that society should make no effort to prolong life beyond that point.

For example, an elderly man in the same hospital ward as

Mrs. Morgan was slipping into a peaceful and quiet death. He had arranged all of his affairs, had made peace with his family, and had welcomed his pastor's last ministrations. He had a readiness to die, feeling that his time had come and that he was slipping into a deep and final sleep—the way he had always hoped to die. But in the middle of the night, as he was dying, a new young resident physician in the hospital, discovered his condition and insisted on connecting him to a respirator. The family protested, asserting that such a decision should be made only by the family doctor, who at the moment was not available. But the young doctor said: "I'm in charge here and no one who is my responsibility is going to die if there is anything I can do to delay or prevent it." What happened the next day would be someone else's responsibility, but tonight he was going to "undertake heroic measures" to save a life. So, over the patient's protests and over the protests of the family, a peaceful and happy death was interrupted for some unnecessary, discomforting and expensive treatment. When one member of the family accused the resident physician of being unkind, he admitted it, saying that the happiness of a patient was not his business. His was by necessity, he said, a rigorous scientific attitude which asserted that a physician must never give up on a patient until every last alternative and possibility of treatment has been pursued to the end.

As for Mrs. Morgan herself, at a late point in her life when she was ready to die and had no more meaningful life ahead of her, she got pneumonia—which would have carried her away into a peaceful death as she wished. But her physician gave her miracle drugs to cure the pneumonia so that she could linger with cancer a few more days.

6. *Dying people have the right to be cared for by professionals who have a positive attitude about palliative care and who are free from taboos and wrong attitudes about death.*

The two belong together. Krant suggests that western society needs to recover a meaningful view of death, perhaps the view of "safe passage" which sees death as a normal stage of life like birth.[8] Within such a perspective a dying person can retain a sense of self-worth, self-control, dignity, and can affirm the right to live fully until the moment of death. Instead of an atmosphere of gloom, such as surrounded Mrs. Morgan, the goal of those who work with terminally-ill persons should be one of seeking to make them comfortable and happy, even giving them pleasure. However one defines the goals for dying persons, questions of attitude and point of view are crucial. For example, the physician should not see death as a personal defeat which therefore must be delayed at the cost of misery to the patient and family. In other words, the patient has the right to a *caring environment* which is possible only if health-care personnel have the right attitude. The dying person has the right to be free from the fear that he or she will be left alone or abandoned—which in fact happened to Mrs. Morgan when she was dying. The dying person of course has the right to sustained, expert medical attention—*i.e.*, a doctor who will continue to see the patient regularly and nurses who are patient, skilled, and understanding. But when doctors and nurses are neglectful—and the evidence shows that Mrs. Morgan was not the only one who gets less attention when dying—the neglect is usually caused by attitudes toward death which are unexamined. Family members, too, may withdraw into feelings of helplessness and despair, sometimes even running away, or at least withdrawing in spirit even though they continue to be physically near to the dying person.

Just before Mrs. Morgan died, a nurse came into her room and tried to remove the small towel she was clutching in her hand. Mrs. Morgan's last words included a protest: "I thought you had abandoned me, too!" Then, fighting to hold onto the towel, she added: "Let me keep it. I'm pretending it is the napkin I've always kept in my trunk, intending to hold as I died." This was the napkin she kept as a souvenir of the night her husband had proposed.

FOR FURTHER READING

Anderson, W. F., "The Elderly at the End of Life," *Nursing Times*, Feb. 8, 1973; Brown, Esther I. *New Dimensions of Patient Care: Patients as People.* New York: Russell Sage Foundation, 1964; Glaser, B. G., *et al. Awareness of Dying.* Chicago: Aldine Press, 1961; Grollman, Earl, *et al. Concerning Death.* Boston: Beacon Press, 1974; Langone, John. *Vital Signs.* Boston: Little, Brown and Co., 1976; Mannes, Marya. *Last Rights.* New York: William Morrow, 1976; Strauss, A. L. and Glaser, B. G. *Anguish: A Case Study of a Dying Trajectory.* Mill Valley, Calif., The Sociology Press, 1970; Twycross, R. C., "The Terminal Care of Patients with Lung Cancer," *Postgraduate Medical Journal,* October, 1973; Wilkes, Eric, "Terminal Care and the Special Nursing Unit," *Nursing Times,* June 9, 1975.

2

The Dilemma of the Family

The problems faced by the members of a family, who stand helplessly by the dying person, not knowing what to say or do, have rarely been given enough study or attention to enable the family to cope with them. Emma, for example, had stayed with Mrs. Morgan day after day, and almost every evening, for week after exhausting week as her mother lay dying. She neglected her own health and her family's until everyone's nerves were ragged with exhaustion. Yet the family exploded with anger when they learned that on the night Mrs. Morgan died Emma had gone home to sleep instead of staying at the hospital with her mother. Their anger was compounded by guilt and ignorance, for the attending physician had ordered Emma to go home and sleep. He had told her that Mrs. Morgan would not die during the night—even though he was sure he was lying—because she herself was becoming a problem at the hospital. In other words, for the sake of the morale and efficiency of the hospital staff, he lied to her in order for her to get some badly-needed rest.

One of the nurses, not knowing that the physician had told Emma to go home, chided her the next day for abandoning her mother at the time of death. At that moment Emma exploded with rage loud enough to be heard all over the hospital ward: "I've tried to do right!" she shouted. "I've done what everyone told me to do and no one has helped me!"

Who should have given more help, support, and guidance to Mrs. Morgan's daughter and to other members of the family? Her clergyman? Emma was a member of a parish in another city, near her own home. Her mother's pastor was new, swamped with an impossible burden of work in an inner-city parish which was understaffed and underfinanced. Nearly every person in the church's community had serious problems, and the new pastor was young and inexperienced in the ways of hospitals. He had been as frustrated over Mrs. Morgan's situation as Emma was, but the pastor tended to defer to the authority of physicians even when he was suspicious of misdiagnosis, mistreatment, and/or neglect. Rather than assuming his role as an equally competent professional who has the responsibility of serving as watchdog over the quality of care given to his people in the hospital, the pastor advised Emma to trust her physician and not question his expertise in pain care. Nor was he willing to challenge hospital rules and procedures when Emma wanted to get her mother moved away from another patient whose moans and screams were making life miserable for Mrs. Morgan. Emma asked him what she should do when she found that the nurses had improper and inadequate instructions from the physician or that one nurse was failing to follow medication instructions properly. Later he had told Emma that it would be impossible to take Mrs. Morgan home for a week end, as her mother was begging for her to do, when in fact it might have been quite feasible.

For a clergyman adequately to advise the family on such matters he would have needed to be well informed on the procedures and possibilities—which were different in each of the several hospitals where he had people—and which in turn meant he was especially dependent upon the counsel and assistance of the hospital chaplaincy. There were part-time Catholic and Protestant chaplains at the hospital, both of whom were at one time or another very attentive to Mrs. Morgan, but neither seemed to be available when Emma needed to talk. Emma and her mother were Anglican, and the Protestant chaplain was on vacation at the most crucial time. He listened to Emma occasionally, and tried to cheer her up, but as a clergyman whose position at the hospital was at best tenuous, he was probably unwilling to challenge the medical professionals whose attitude toward him seemed to be one of tolerance so long as he didn't stick his nose into their business. For he was aware of a good deal of sloppy work around the hospital— such as many cases of the wrong pills being given—but did not feel it was his business to point the facts out. He admitted later that it was apparent from the beginning that Mrs. Morgan had been placed in the wrong hospital, but it was not his business to discuss that fact nor attempt to deal with it, once it was an accomplished fact.

The social worker at the hospital was part-time and incompetent. She gave Emma incorrect information about rules and possibilities, and advised Emma to "trust the doctors and nurses who know more about things than you do," when in fact Emma was realizing that her mother's case was being seriously mismanaged. Of course, Emma had lots of advice and opinions from neighbors, friends, and members of the family— all of whom disagreed. With inadequate support and help, Emma resolutely made up her mind that she had no choice except to do what she thought was right—that is, to rely completely on the physician and do whatever he recommended. She was quite bitter, therefore, when, after the funeral, she was confronted with stories from other people who had experienced that physician's neglect and incompetence, and especially from persons who said: "I tried to tell you!" Indeed, she said, everyone had tried to "tell her." She had heard one thing from the social worker, another from the chaplain, and different things from nurses and families of other patients. Not even members of the hospital staff seemed to have conferred with each other so as to agree on their advice to her, to help Emma sort out the truth as she was incompetent to do alone. The one thing everyone seemed to say was "rely on the doctor." Emma shared with other members of her family an overwhelming sense of helplessness, and she felt numb because of her feelings of guilt over not having been willing or able to keep her mother at home. Lamerton found that social workers sometimes neglect a dying patient in order to help members of the family,[1] but Emma's problem was exactly the opposite. The social worker devoted a good deal of time to talking with Mrs. Morgan to find out why she cried all the time, and because Mrs. Morgan was blind. All she did for Emma was increase her guilt by saying: "If you don't like the way things are done in the hospital, why don't you take your mother home and care for her there."

Problems of Home Care

Why, in fact, did Mrs. Morgan's daughter feel that she could not continue to take care of her mother at home? Well, for one thing, home care was exhausting. A visiting nurse came to provide needed help; but by the time the nurse had made her first visit, Emma was already exhausted and convinced she could not cope alone. Also, the visiting nurse was not available in the middle of the night, or on call at the times Emma needed her most—as, for example, the time Mrs. Morgan fell out of bed at three o'clock in the morning and was too heavy for Emma to help back into bed alone. Emma was exhausted because she did not have any days off, not even enough hours to sleep much of the time. Other members of the family were undependable for any real help, and in any case lacked skill and self-confidence. The visiting nurse was helpful at this point. She taught Emma how to make a bed with a patient in it, how to give her mother a bath, and give her medication, and so on. But the family needed more than simple instruction, the members needed help on call and needed counseling on their attitudes toward death itself. Despite all the real problems which Mrs. Morgan's family faced in trying to take care of her at home, the central difficulty revolved around their view of life and death. In the view of those loved ones closest to Mrs. Morgan, death was something to be dreaded and feared. Their attitudes contributed to the negative environment surrounding her, regardless of whether she was at home or in a facility. After Mrs. Morgan's death Emma finally came to see that if her attitude had been different she probably could have cared for her mother at home. She admitted that she was so fearful of how to handle death when it came; she so dreaded the possibility of being at home alone with her mother at the time of death that she was not prepared to take advantage of the possibilities for help that were open to her through visiting nurses and other assistance. She certainly had not been aggressive in seeking out other resources in the community, nor had it occurred to her that counseling was one of her main needs.

As in so many human situations, most of the basic difficulties could have been resolved had there been better communication among the persons involved. Mrs. Morgan's family did not understand some very simple things: the fact that it would be possible for her to be comfortable with palliative care and find some measure of enjoyment at the end of her life, and that her last days could be seen as a time of fulfillment and completion for her life, and not merely as a troublesome period of survival to be endured.[2] Mrs. Morgan, in her own way— unfortunately not adequately shared with her family, since perhaps she considered it a private matter—had a plan for her time of dying. She wanted to spend her last hours reflecting upon the meaning of her life, summing it up as she looked a last time at each of her most meaningful souvenirs. Although her family was dimly aware of her intentions and wishes, they lacked the point of view which would see the value of her quest for meaning and thus make it possible for them to help her. This also made it difficult for them to care for her at home.

It is clear that it is not necessarily true that health-care professionals are the best persons to meet the emotional and the psychological needs of dying persons and their families, or at least not without special preparation. Mrs. Morgan's physician, indeed, may have had as limited a view of the meaning of life and death as did Mrs. Morgan's family. Nor is it clear that any one source of counseling was adequately available to the family, so far as they knew, nor did the various persons who counseled them consult with one another and make sure that adequate counseling was undertaken by someone who was prepared for the task by education and experience. Emma might have been more willing and able to take care of her mother at home had she not recently shared the trauma of her neighbors, the Klines, who had tried to care for a dying youngster at home because the child had been so miserable and unhappy in the hospital. A number of the problems which the Klines had faced reminded Emma of her total feelings of inadequacy at the time of her father's death. Even worse, for example, when Timmy Kline died, the family had been unable to find a physician who would come to the house and there was even greater trauma over the problem of delay in getting the death certificate signed and the body removed from the home. The Klines had lost touch with other physicians during the year Timmy was in the hospital, and after taking him home they called the hospital to ask for the help of the physician who had attended Timmy there, only to be told that they should have made arrangements with a doctor in their community. That experience recalled vividly back into Emma's mind what the answering service had told her when she had phoned the substitute doctor (her own physician was out of town) about her father's death: "But surely doctor told you that he doesn't make house calls." The answering-service operator was subsequently reprimanded, but the memory served to confirm Emma's judgment that Mrs. Morgan had to go to the hospital and stay there where she would have 24-hour-a-day care, with pain control, physicians always available, and where the staff took responsibility for such matters as signing death certificates.

Family Needs

Some of the rights outlined for patients also apply to the families of patients, including the right to be heard, the right to be told all the facts, the right to share in decision-making along with physicians, the right to keep control of their own lives insofar as possible . . . and not have life traumatically interrupted over long periods of illness. But needs are even more fundamental than rights. What family needs are suggested by reflection upon this case study of Mrs. Morgan and her family?

1. *A family needs counseling.*

The family of a cancer patient, for example, needs counseling about cancer itself—not only after a member of the family is terminally ill but also in nearly all situations. One physician has said that more consideration needs to be given to the "needs of the vast numbers of cancer treated patients who for a number of years live with the fear of recurrence. . . . the medical profession can be criticized here, as well as in the terminal patient care area, for failure to give patient *and* family enough continuing support whenever cancer occurs, recurs, or is a worry, as well as when it becomes terminal." [3]

David K. Wellisch, Ph.D., of the University of California at Los Angeles, told the 1976 Annual Meeting of the American Society of Clinical Oncology about a multiple family therapy group program for cancer patients and their families.[4] For the first seven months of the program, which was directed by a clinical psychologist, the cancer patients themselves did not attend the sessions, and family members attended only as they felt the need. Since family members often expressed emotions of rage, sadness, fear, and/or guilt, the planners of the program felt that patients would be overwhelmed, but this was found not to be the case. Attendance improved and the effectiveness of the program increased when patients also began to attend. The purpose of the program was to help each family attain maximal intimacy, sharing, and support, as well as to deal with the eventual death of the family member. The group meetings tended to focus, Wellisch said, on "maximal utilization of remaining life, rather than upon death." Often these weekly sessions were the only social life of some persons who had very sick relatives. Although physicians did not attend the sessions—this was so that families would feel free to express possible emotions of anger toward the physicians—they noted a much greater openness between themselves and the persons who attended the sessions, and tended to feel that they had a better relationship with the families. This carried over even to those families that did not participate, but who knew that the sessions were available through the cooperation of the physician. The advantage of the group process for families of terminally-ill persons was perhaps most evidenced by the ability of members of participating families to confront each other— they tended to be less tolerant of anyone's resistance than the therapists were. Such a group session would undoubtedly have facilitated a badly needed conversation not only among members of Mrs. Morgan's family but also with her.

2. *A family needs information.*

Another basic family need, and perhaps the most important one, is for information. One study comparing cancer and surgical patients found that "only a small proportion of the physicians" provided their patients with tangible, explicit information.[5] Cancer patients and their families, even more than others, perceive significant conflicts and disagreements among their various sources of information. Some of their anxiety may have been caused not only by the lack of adequate information but also by the fact that persons they talked with disagreed—as was certainly the case with Mrs. Morgan's family.

People become aware of inconsistencies in what they are told by physicians and other health-care persons involved. The study concluded that the more ambiguity which the patients face, the more difficult the problem they will have in coping: "There is a direct relationship between the anxieties of cancer patients and the multiple contradictions and misleading information they are given." The information Mrs. Morgan's family needed was not just the facts about her illness. They needed to know more about many things: alternatives for her care; that there was a difference between the two hospitals she might have entered; that there were other nursing homes which would have been better places for her; that there were ways to appeal for help when they discovered the hospital staff doctors and nurses were not functioning properly; that more and different help was available from the visiting nurse and other community agencies.

Possible Alternatives

There were plenty of agencies ready to give Emma a sympathetic listening ear and some psychological support. But just as Mrs. Morgan's fundamental need—which must not be overlooked—was for excellence in medical care, so, also, Emma's need, in order to care for her mother at home, was for help, not sympathy. The family tried to employ help to take care of Mrs. Morgan at home. Perhaps it did not work out because the family members lacked proper advice as to where and how to find the right help—but it is quite as probable that the help was not available. One pastor in the community said that within his own congregation there were at least twenty elderly people who needed to employ someone to help them if they were to remain in their homes, and he had not been able to find competent persons who were available. The community did not even have one of the rather expensive professional home-care aid services.

The family tried a nursing home and again had a bad experience, again perhaps because they lacked guidance and help in finding the right one for Mrs. Morgan. But, truth to tell, the right sort of nursing home to take care of a terminally-ill person may not exist in a community. It was apparently the policy of the best nursing homes in the area not to accept terminally-ill people, and to send their own patients to hospitals when they became terminally ill. At the same time the hospitals in the community had a policy of dismissing terminally-ill people in order to provide beds for persons who could be cured. To families who felt they could not take care of a dying patient at home these hospitals recommended that they look for a nursing home! When this contradiction was pointed out to them, hospital and nursing home officials all expressed surprise at learning the policy of the other. The nursing home that Mrs. Morgan's family finally found, and which was willing to take her, was not the best. Indeed, it operated on the policy of "benign neglect," which has been described as "taking the same care of elderly people that you would do at home." Emma said that this was true: "I couldn't manage her at home and they couldn't manage her at the nursing home!"

Aftereffects

Moving her mother to the hospital did not give Emma the rest she wanted and needed. The truth was, she put down a heavy burden and picked up two others which turned out to be worse than anticipated. She had known it would be tiresome and difficult to commute back and forth from the hospital—spending at least eight hours a week in her car. But she had not anticipated the burden of worry and guilt. Her mother's death thus came as no surprise or shock after so many months of lingering so near death. Indeed, it came almost as a relief to Emma that she could quit worrying and running back and forth to the hospital—all the while suffering pangs of guilt for not going more often. Everyone complimented her on how well she bore her grief and kept control of herself at the funeral and the weeks afterward. Then, as the burden of her guilt grew, Emma began to fall to pieces. No one had helped to prepare her for the bereavement process before or after her mother's death. The crisis became especially acute when she began to sort out and dispose of the "junk" her mother had accumulated at home. As she went through the photograph albums and scrapbooks she began to realize what her mother had wanted in her last weeks and how cruel everyone had been to refuse the souvenirs to her. One day a neighbor found her in hysterics.

Dr. Colin Murray Parkes has studied the shock that comes into the lives of many grieving persons who are not given adequate help in understanding their feelings and needs.[6] In his interviews with widows he found many persons like Emma who felt betrayed by their physicians. It was only human, of course, for Emma to search for someone else to blame—her children, doctors, nurses, her pastor—for it was difficult for her to deal with her own feelings of guilt, her self-punishment and self-blame. Emma began to withdraw from life as an old person herself, spending disorganized days weeping over her mother's scrapbooks. The numbness which had protected and isolated her at the funeral and afterward now turned to loneliness and despair. She began to suspect that she had symptoms which indicated she would follow her mother with the same type of terminal illness. Her children began to avoid her—as at times they had avoided their grandmother—because they could neither understand nor sympathize with her weeping and complaining. Emma would rehearse over and over her feelings of guilt: "If only we had taken her this one scrapbook," or "We could have brought a few of her things to the hospital, different items each time we visited her."

Her mother's pastor tried to help by visiting her several times, but Emma would not listen to him nor to her mother's physician because of intense feelings of self-blame which she associated with them. She needed the help of a psychiatrist to interpret the whole process of bereavement, as well as his help to deal with her other emotional problems, but she would not hear of it. "All I want," she shouted at her sons, "is to be left alone." So her family and neighbors increasingly left her alone —another victim of society's ineptness in dealing with death and the dying, as well as the bereavement and other attendant problems of the families of terminally-ill persons.

The Hospice Alternative

How different would the experience of Mrs. Morgan and her family have been had she gone to a hospice or to a hospital with a hospice team and program? Emma's experience provides an interesting contrast to that of a woman we will here call Mrs. Green, the wife of a musician whose dying days were radically improved by the intervention of a hospice team. "I cried when he was sick, especially when not enough was being done about his terrible pain," Mrs. Green said. "So at the memorial service I was able to enjoy memories, even to enjoy with him the music his friends played for him, that they had so often before played with him."

Mr. Green had his first operation in 1973, after a long period of refusing to tell others of his pain. He had never had much use for physicians and hospitals, and the thirty-four days of tests, operations, and postoperative treatment of his ulcerated tumor confirmed his worst fears. He went home for a year and a half of intensive life, performing for small groups, playing at churches, until August of 1975 when his suffering grew unbearable. In September of 1975 he returned to the hospital for more tests, and his doctor decided there was little they could do for him. His pain and misery grew worse, especially because of his inability to move his bowels, until January of 1976 when Mr. Green was again admitted to the hospital for the last time. The doctors felt he would soon die, but he took an unexpected turn for the better and wanted his music and his records. He wanted to play a pipe organ. Not much else had meaning for him in his severe pain.

What were his wife's emotions? In 1973 after the first operation she was told that he might live five years, but it might be only six months. She sorrowed at the prospect that their good life together—they both loved music—was soon to end, but she suffered most because of his terrible pain. In some ways, she said, it was worse seeing one she loved in that kind of pain than it would have been to bear the pain herself. "What troubled me most, of course," she said, "was that I could do nothing to help him. There was nothing I could say or do when his pride would not allow him to ask for pain medicine. I tried to tell the nurses to give it to him anyway, as the physician had instructed, but the doctor was busy and didn't come around often. The nurses simply couldn't believe his pain was so bad when he said nothing. They couldn't read his expression as I could."

Mrs. Green gave up her home, thirty miles from the hospital, to rent an apartment around the corner when it became clear to her that he would never leave the hospital. She knew she must conserve the strength she was dissipating in travel, but she did not know where to turn for the help she needed. She saw that the various health-care professionals who were working with her husband needed to coordinate their efforts, but, an uninformed lay person, she was not heard, nor did she know how or what to say. She needed more information about pain control and the various alternatives for better care for her dying husband; but where could she turn in a situation where the physicians made crucial decisions without discussing the possible alternatives with her? Fortunately, her doctor recognized that he was busy and could do little for Mr. Green or his wife. Then he became aware of a new possibility for them. He turned the Greens over to the hospice team which was beginning to function in the hospital.

When the hospice nurse, who was specially trained to work

with the terminally ill, first came to see Mr. Green she found him so weak that he could not pick up the telephone, his weakness being partly the result of the great strain involved in his effort to hide his suffering from his wife and from the nurses. The hospice nurse found that Mr. Green had been so successful that the floor nurses believed his pain was not very great at all. They were, in any case, trained to withhold pain-killing drugs until the patient asked for them, and in his pride Mr. Green never asked, thinking it more manly to bear and hide his suffering.

The aim of the hospice team was to make Mr. Green's life pleasant and comfortable so long as he survived. Therefore, they immediately explained to him what the pain was doing to his strength and to his wife's morale. Once he realized that his wife was fully aware of his pain, he readily welcomed the hospice team's medication to control his pain. He was kept free of pain as the medication was given before he began to suffer. Once he was free from pain it was possible to control the other symptoms and to build up his strength and morale. The style of treatment was radically different from what the hospital would do if it were thought that he could be cured, or if the main emphasis was on keeping him alive on any terms. The hospice team ministered to his wife as much as to the husband to nurture and enrich their life together, to help them grow closer in their last weeks together. The team helped him to discover other meanings of courage than just a stoic bearing of pain. One day the hospice nurse asked: "What can we do to make you more comfortable?" And Mr. Green replied: "Give me no more needles." So they arranged for him to get his medication in the form of pills or suppositories. Mr. Green then found it possible to be more open and communicative with everyone around him, at the same time developing a new appreciation for the skill, dedication, and humanity of the floor nurses and resident medical staff.

Since the hospice program was new in the hospital, one of

the team's jobs was to re-educate the nurses and floor staff by demonstrating the new ways of caring for terminally-ill people like Mr. Green. They did not therefore take over from the nurses in charge, but offered to give them help in carrying their heavy load. In the presence of the other staff they explained to Mrs. Green the evidence that her husband was suffering more than had been noted—which of course Mrs. Green already knew, but it educated the floor staff without embarrassing them or suggesting they didn't know. Armed with Mr. Green's charts since 1973, including information about all the medication he had had or which had been prescribed, the team explained to Mrs. Green the kind of pain control that was possible for him and told her that the hospice team would be available to her at any hour of the day or night if she had questions or problems. If some question bothered her in the middle of the night she was to feel free to telephone the team members' homes if necessary.

"They did much more for us than just make him free from pain and more comfortable," Mrs. Green explained. "The second hospice nurse to come to talk to him began by asking what his interests were, what he enjoyed in life. Happily, she was a musician too. He told her of his wish to play an organ again, so she took him to the hospital chapel and let him play. Next, she worked with him in preparing a musical program for other patients. She sang and he accompanied her. His fingers wouldn't behave right and at points he became confused as he played, but that didn't matter as it had the last time he tried to play in a church. His favorite type of social evening had always been to play music with a group of friends and this was how he saw his musical program at the hospital. As a result of this sharing of music, which represented so much of the meaning of his life, the hospital became for him a more human place, whereas before he had described it as a sort of massive incubator where the human touch was replaced by technology. When his wife arrived in the morning she now found him with a big smile on his face, his eyes bright, listening to his favorite classical music on an FM radio or his record player. Instead of dealing with first one impersonal nurse and then another; instead of Mrs. Green being resentful that the nurses were not doing what she thought they should do to control his pain—both of the Greens began to feel that the floor staff were their friends, whose aim was not merely to help Mr. Green live, but to help him live well.

The hospice staff helped Mrs. Green to understand that many of the nurses, well educated as they were and with all the right attitudes in principle, had never before had adequate experience with dying persons and that instead of resenting any mistakes or limitations they might have, she could see herself as learning with them—even in part becoming one of their teachers, to help them learn what the emotions, problems, and thoughts of the wife of a terminally-ill patient were. Mrs. Green said that the chaplain on the hospice team was very helpful. He realized that she had pains and needs herself, which had to be exposed and managed. She had not noticed that her own problems were an added burden to her husband, who saw what she tried to hide as clearly as she had seen the pain he had tried to conceal. "The chaplain talked to us together," she said. "And to me alone as much as was necessary for me to unload my burden of guilt and worry. The chaplain was most helpful with the grief process, beginning long before my husband died. I think of the chaplain as a tall, strength-giving person when actually he has a rather small physical frame, although he is large in spirit. He helped me cry, not that I hadn't wept each night at home, hiding my face under the covers to do what I never allowed myself to do in my husband's presence. The chaplain and the psychiatrist helped my husband and me to have natural tears together, tears we really enjoyed. It was good for us to be able to comfort each other more openly after trying for so long to hide our grief from each other. Does it sound wrong for me to say that my husband and

I actually enjoyed sharing together our grief over his coming death? Because of our being able to cry together it has been so much easier for me to manage my grief and get on with life now that he is gone."

Mrs. Green said that she is lonesome for her husband of course, now that he is dead, but she is able to sleep well, knowing that he is no longer in pain. This is, in part, because she was able to sleep well even before he died, once the hospice team was helping both of them. She had been unable to eat, was losing weight, and was perilously close to becoming ill herself, but the team helped her to build up her psychic and physical strength so that she was better prepared to stand up under the impact of his death, funeral, and the grief she found she now had strength to share. By contrast, Dr. Parkes' studies of wives in bereavement have discovered a very unhealthy morbidity and much earlier mortality on the part of grieving spouses in cases where there was no adequate bereavement preparation and care program.[7]

Mrs. Green is now working as a volunteer in the hospice. "The hospice program," she tells the families of other dying patients, "gave my husband a reason and a chance to die like a man and gave me the opportunity to live better with him as he was dying." She has kept her apartment near the hospital and especially likes to visit and work with dying patients who lack a family or whose families have especially difficult problems. She is able to understand and to interpret to others the necessity, as she puts it, of fighting for your loved ones. "But it is important to know what to fight. I was, as many families do, falling into the error of seeing the hospital staff as the enemy; especially when one of the nurses objected to giving my dying husband the full dose of narcotics he needed because he might become addicted. And I was too absorbed with my own problems to see how busy the floor nurse was, with five beds to a room and so many rooms to care for. The hospice staff not only became my allies in the struggle to help my husband have a happy end to his life but they also helped me to see all the hospital staff as the allies they should be. Together we were helped to move into a healthier, more adequate view of death and its meaning. The hospice psychiatrist, who helped me work out my feelings of resentment toward the staff nurses and doctors, also helped them work out their feelings of resentment toward me and the way I had continually tried to interfere with their work. My emotions were freed up so I could be more supportive and understanding of the staff, and could therefore devote myself positively to my husband. But they were helped, too, and needed the hospice team for information, point of view, and support in doing actual work when the situation got rough."

In contrast to Mrs. Morgan and Emma's experience, the hospice social worker seemed to know exactly the right time to offer help to Mrs. Green with a wide variety of legal bureaucratic matters before Mr. Green died and afterward. She helped with funeral arrangements and financial advice. At one point, when Mr. and Mrs. Green were out in the hospital garden with the social worker, she explored with them the possibility of Mr. Green going home for a week-end visit, with various helpers available to make it possible. Mr. Green died before the arrangements were completed, but he greatly enjoyed making the plans and the anticipation of going home to die. Always a person who loved to make plans, it gave him something positive to look forward to during his last days. Mrs. Green also could relax and enjoy the idea, secure in the knowledge that the hospital pharmacy, clinic, home-care nurses, the social worker, and others would guarantee to her all the help and support she would need to take him home.

Planning for Better Care

Rather than proposing abstract theories and schemes, the health-care professionals and the others who are planning and developing such hospice programs have carefully examined the experience of specific persons, such as Mrs. Morgan, Mrs. Green, and their families. The hospice philosophy, which sees the patient-*and*-family as the unit of care, rather than just the patient alone, has emerged from experience in dealing with large numbers of terminally-ill persons. This has implications for many other aspects of health care, but is especially crucial for the dying and·their families as the cases in this chapter have illustrated. Those who have been responsible for planning and research at the New Haven Hospice program, for example, see their work as providing a demonstration model where health-care professionals can come to see how this type of care—combining, as it does, excellence in scientific medical and nursing skills with reverence for life and its spirit —increases the capacity of terminally-ill patients and their families to live through the period of trauma with tranquillity and dignity, with the help of a staff specially trained and experienced in helping patient and family relieve their distress.[8] Rather than ask patients and families with their varied life-styles to adjust to the unyielding regimen of the hospital, the hospice staff and planners have seen that families could be helped to retain their integrity and life-styles, with the hospice program adapted to their needs rather than vice versa. The patient and family are encouraged by the hospice staff and its philosophy to assume active roles in decision-making and in determining the quality of life during the period of terminal illness. Patients and families become teachers of other patients and families, as they share their experience, and even help the medical staff itself to become more understanding and helpful during the time of crisis which all share at death. Families and others involved with terminally-ill persons expend a tremendous amount of energy and "this needs replenishment."[9] Patients and families can help with this replenishment by a "hospice family" whose members come and go, wherein both strong and weak, giver and receiver, skilled and medically unskilled, all work together to strengthen one another.

A hospice program, therefore, can actually succeed in keeping family members together, rather than divided and in conflict as in Mrs. Morgan's case. It can help them become skilled members of the "caring team" as it trains family members to participate in treatment and provides for them the skilled assistance they need to teach each other and to work together. The hospice concept, for example, sees it as important for families to continue cooking favorite foods for a patient—even for a terminally-ill person in a medical facility—to stimulate the appetite and keep up the morale of the patient, especially one from an ethnic group whose special food is very important to the patient. And regardless of whether the hospice provides a special facility to replace hospital or nursing home or whether the hospice team functions within a hospital or simply as a home-care program, all of the services a family needs can be provided, including the best possible medical care, bereavement care, special social and educational programs for family *and* patient, and whatever else is needed.

FOR FURTHER READING

Branson, Helen K., "The Terminal Patient and His Family," *Bedside Patient*, June 1970; Gerber, Irwin, *et al.*, "Anticipating Grief in Widows and Widowers," *Journal of Gerontology*, Vol. 30, no. 2, March 1975; Eyers, Saul, "Effect of Death on the Living," *Journal of Practical Nursing*, Jan. 1975; Pincus, Lily, *Death and the Family*. New York: Pantheon, 1975; Schoenberg, E., *et al.*, *Loss and Grief*. New York: Columbia University Press, 1970; and for suggestive procedures for working with family groups, see Schwartz, Marc, "Situation/Transition Groups: A Conceptualization and Review," *American Journal of Orthopsychiatry*, Vol. 45, no. 5, Oct. 1975.

Health-Care Professionals
and the Dying

Physicians, nurses, and others who work with dying persons need understanding and appreciative support, even as at the same time they must accept some criticism and blame for their unrealistic expectations. A book like this which proposes needed changes may seem at points to be negative toward health-care professionals, but physicians themselves are the source of most of the negative criticism included here. This is as it should be, for much of the medical profession's progress has depended upon an ability to criticize itself in order to upgrade its performance. In being critical of the care of some cancer patients, therefore, that criticism should be taken in the context of progress made which has resulted in over half of cancer patients being cured in our contemporary society. The hospital environment is often a miserable place for the terminally ill, however, precisely because it is an institution designed for cure and is staffed by physicians and others whose passionate devotion to cure has been one of the foundations for the great strides which have been made.

Those who have hope of returning to productive life and work are willing to put up with hospital miseries which they see as perhaps needed to guarantee the efficiency and effectiveness of cure. But once a patient has no more hope for cure, a person like Mrs. Morgan—too often relegated to a dark room at the end of the hospital corridor as an embarrassing failure to be kept out of sight—finds the regime designed for cure to be dehumanizing. The phenomenon is increasingly studied, but there are clearer insights into what the problem is than in what to do about it or how to do it. The problem is complex.

The World of the Hospital

Dr. Melvin Krant, for example, points out the ironic fact that the "strange world" of the hospital was originally established to administer to the sufferings of *persons*, but now the medical staff has become increasingly concerned with *disease*, even to the extent of forgetting about or losing sight of the needs and wishes of the patients.[1] Almost unintentionally sometimes, but deliberately in many other cases because of the pressure of overwhelming work, an "impersonal professional style" seems to have replaced the human personal concern and relationship which has so long been an important tool of the physician in accomplishing his work. No matter what attention is given to architectural styles and paint colors, the environment of the hospital is created by the attitudes of the persons who work there. It is characteristic of nearly all of society's institutions that they tend to become self-serving, often to the extent of losing sight of the needs of the persons they were established to serve. Many a school, for example, tends to organize itself to serve the needs of the teachers rather than the needs of the pupils, just as many hospitals are poor places for dying persons because they are organized to serve the needs of the staff rather than those of the patients.

Institutional pride leads many hospitals to the necessity for exorbitant rate increases because they compete with other hospitals in the purchase of expensive medical equipment —some of which could undoubtedly be shared if hospitals planned to cooperate. Since 1950 the cost of keeping a dying person in the hospital for one day has risen by 500 per cent.[2] Much of this equipment, two thirds of which is obsolete within less than ten years, is not needed at all by terminally-ill persons, who nevertheless have their per-day bed charges increased to help pay for it. Of course it is not easy to sort out the hospital administrator's need for success in creating a great institution from the needs of ill persons in the hospital. But when asked if hospitals or nursing homes couldn't function everywhere with the hospice point of view and program for terminally-ill people, the hospital chaplain who is chairman of the New Haven Hospice Board replied: "In many cases, Yes. But there is a psychological advantage to taking the dying person away from the noises and antiseptic smells of the hospital, which is organized to facilitate cure by the most efficient means possible." No longer in need of expensive curative treatments, the terminally-ill person instead needs a warm, comfortable, homey, pleasant environment. The attending physician and the hospital directors have no interest in turning the hospital into a luxury hotel for the comfort of patients, but they could give more attention to the scientific laboratory atmosphere of "noises and antiseptic smells" and unexamined procedures and assumptions—all of which result in an impersonal style of care, in an acceptance of the fact that for some persons the hospital is just a dumping ground, with the only responsibility of the institution being to keep the patient's body functioning, and that it is better to spend money on equipment than on care to enhance the quality of life.

What changes are needed in the attitudes and procedures of physicians and nurses, for example, if a more adequate and humane environment is to be maintained for dying persons? Before turning to the challenge which the hospice concept is making to the idea that death is a defeat for the physician, and to the notion that the dying must be kept in a sterile, intensive-care atmosphere long after there is no possibility of cure, let us view the situation again from Mrs. Morgan's perspective.

Mrs. Morgan and the Physicians

Mrs. Morgan had been quite satisfied with her family doctor, a friend and professional health-care provider, for a number of years. He had given her more than adequate attention and care as long as he felt that there was something he could do. But once it was clear that she was going to die, he seemed to lose interest. Perhaps he felt that his time belonged to persons whom he could help. He explained to her family that he had turned her over to specialists who could do more for her than he could. He came to see her less often, stopping by only briefly from time to time, and brushed off her complaints and tears with the no longer comforting words that "everyone is doing everything he can." As for the specialists, neither Mrs. Morgan nor her family could determine, especially in the last weeks of her life, just which physician or physicians were giving the instructions and making the decisions. In retrospect it seems clear that at times no one was—each doctor was perhaps assuming that someone else was responsible. It is quite possible, also, that all of them were in a sense running away from the face of death. The fact is that none of them—and this includes the young inexperienced nurses who were caring for Mrs. Morgan—had had adequate instruction in the best methods of caring for terminally-ill persons. Medical schools are now giving more attention to death and dying as a subject of study, but the fact is that the issue is a philosophical and psychological bundle which cannnot easily be resolved by a theoretical course. Society shaped the medical and nursing students into persons whose attitudes and characters cannot easily be changed, long before they began professional training.

David Duncombe and Chase Kimball, for example, have been examining the psychological needs of medical students, and psychological factors which played an important part in their decision to become physicians.[3] Medicine is attractive to many medical students because of its precision and predict bility, and this type of personality tends to become frustrated with those aspects of medicine which can't be predicted and where knowledge is uncertain or research is as yet inadequate' for decision-making. These persons tend therefore to concentrate their attention in areas where they have control and to avoid other areas of frustration and failure—such as death. At the same time, Duncombe and Kimball find that a high percentage of medical students had a death in the family prior to deciding to go to medical school. Most of those students reported the experience to have been "very painful" and with emotions still lingering, although they do not feel that this influenced their decision to become physicians. Duncombe and Kimball, however, feel that medicine is, at least in part, chosen as a way to cope with these experiences. Perhaps also there is an anticipation of the medical student's own death, "a fantasy to control or avoid their own deaths through the 'holy grail' of the miracle cure." Attitudes toward death which may cause a physician almost unconsciously to avoid or treat impersonally his dying patients cannot easily be resolved through a medical school's theoretical course.

Again, a physician's orientation may be so passionately and idealistically directed to curing people that he sees death as a defeat which he wants to avoid at all costs—even sometimes by running away psychologically. Krant reminds us that there is an increasing tendency to treat old age and normal dying as if it were an illness instead of a normal process.[4] This is related to a shift in the attitudes of some medical personnel away from training persons to take care of themselves, to keep in good health through exercise, health habits, clean water, a good diet, toward an attempt to maintain health through use of drugs designed to cure anything. Unfortunately, nurses and physicians get their satisfactions largely from the results they can see—as when a sick person gets back on his feet and is restored to his work—rather from preventive health-care procedures. Financial rewards, too, come to the physician from cures rather than from prevention or from the care of the aged and dying. Psychologically, as long as physicians view death as a defeat—with no doctor wanting to take blame for the failure —they cannot accept dying as a normal human event which requires them to make the last weeks and days of the terminally-ill patient as happy and meaningful as possible. As the medical system is presently constituted, there is no procedure for rewarding a nurse or physician for compassion, but only for science.

Mrs. Morgan, therefore, was made continually to feel that she was a bother, that people were busy, so that she should not ask the hospital staff for attention and care. Perhaps, indeed, the large number of patients in that sort of hospital requires mass treatment with efficiency, but a busy attitude, as Mrs. Morgan herself perceptively noted, is in itself frequently a style of avoidance. Such avoidance on the part of physicians may be compounded of many elements. Even the much discussed question of what to tell a dying patient is in many cases complicated by the physician's lack of communication skill. Some physicians also have a bad conscience about failure or about the sometimes rather shabby use of terminally-ill persons as guinea pigs for medical experimentation. But for many the problem is basically a philosophical one: the lack of an adequate point of view toward death and dying which is rooted in real experience with dying persons, and which has been reflected upon and evaluated through shared discussions with persons who have a more adequate perspective on the meaning of death. While Mrs. Morgan herself, for example, tended to see the universe as good, and death as a good and healthy climax to life, one of her passing specialists made it clear to her that he considered death an evil aspect of an evil universe which he felt called to fight, defy, and oppose to his last breath. Therefore, by daring to die, and by accepting her death, she was becoming as one with the enemy. Drugs, he said, were causing her to relax her fight against death, and pain was something she needed to remind her of the need for vigilance against the "great enemy." In another, similar, situation a nurse said to a physician that her specialty was "people, not tumors," in trying to explain her concern with enhancing the lives of cancer patients. The doctor objected, replying: "But they're all dying! We have a few breasts and colons here, but mostly metastases [where cancer is spreading throughout the body]. It's a very rough world." [5] In other words, he was saying why bother with people who are dying. His concern was with the disease.

"When I was very young," Mrs. Morgan's daughter said, "we had a family doctor who told us that love was the most important part of curing. Nowadays there is no love, not even a personal concern—certainly those young doctors seemed to care more for their machines than for their people." In another hospital it was reported that "the doctor on the floor assumes he does not in fact need a team approach, [for] . . . more personalized patient care, but only tolerates it. The implication is that, as in many acute-care complexes, the emphasis on curative treatment is at odds with individualized, supportive care." [6] Further, the care of terminally-ill cancer patients in this large hospital was reported to be largely the responsibility of fourth-year residents on clinical rotation, who not only lacked experience with death and dying, but who as students were "more interested in the technical and scientific facets of disease progression" than in becoming involved with persons who have emotions and human needs.

Krant suggests that much more attention needs to be given not merely to patients' rights but to the creation of "mutual confidence and trust between patient and physician that allows the sick to feel that all that could be done has been done." [7] This also helps the dying patient to feel that the hospital was established for the patients, not the doctors. According to Krant, it will be far from easy for the medical profession to allow persons to die peacefully and in control of their own lives, for this will require a new approach—a new design for legitimatizing death which can allow for healthy consolation, support and comfort for all dying persons in contrast to the present all-too-frequent concern for prolonging life at any cost.

Mrs. Morgan and the Nurses

Mrs. Morgan's feeling that the "busyness" on her hospital ward was a style of avoidance was not entirely justified, for, after her mother's death, Emma learned that the terminal-care unit at the hospital was seriously, even dangerously, understaffed. It almost seemed as if the hospital administration felt that since little more could be done to cure dying persons, the most able and competent nurses should devote their time to persons who could be restored to health. To Mrs. Morgan's floor was assigned the youngest, least experienced, and sometimes even transient, nurses. Few of these young nurses had sufficient previous experience with death. No attention was given to the emotional needs of these nurses when patients died for whom they had developed some affection and concern. Therefore, to protect themselves, many of the nurses tended to discipline themselves "not to care," to be as aloof as possible toward dying persons, since they were just too overworked to deal with grief.

A patient like Mrs. Morgan, caught up in her own pain and misery, had no perspective from which to view the problem of the young nurses, although her daughter said that some of the other patients on the floor did come to understand and actually tried to help some of the young nurses retain their aloofness. The hospital chaplain said that he was concerned about the feelings of guilt and the distaste which some of the nurses felt for the work in which they were engaged, so that at one point he had gone to the hospital administration to ask for psychiatric help for the nurses dealing with terminally-ill patients. But no funds were available for such support, and the chaplain himself lacked the skill, time, and a position of prestige in the hospital from which to deal with the problem himself. He did try to take time to listen to nurses who needed to talk, but the best advice he could give them was to "get out of there as soon as you can." Physicians tended to give the same advice to the young nurses when they complained. Without deliberate intent, therefore, the hospital administration experienced a large turnover of nurses working with the terminally-ill—a turnover which was too frequent to make it a valuable training experience for anyone. No nurse stayed with dying persons long enough to get the background and experience necessary to develop some expertise along with a point of view to share with new young nurses assigned to the floor.

No wonder that Mrs. Morgan, who in addition was nearly blind, found it difficult to distinguish any one nurse or person on the floor who was concerned with her personally. David Mechanic has pointed out how the heavy work load of the physician makes it difficult for him to give a high priority to meeting psychological and social needs of patients, and therefore relegates such responsibilities to the nurses.[8] But the nurses are equally busy and often face a hospital policy of rotating assignments which makes it exceedingly difficult for a nurse to establish an on-going personal relationship with a patient even under the best circumstances. One observer of a terminal-care ward, whose experiences there demonstrated to him that "human involvement is . . . an essential ingredient in complete terminal care," noted that only the volunteers "of which there were few . . . had time to sit and talk with the patients."[9] Observers studying floor procedures also have found that nurses generally take twice as long to respond to the call bell of a terminal patient as to that of a patient who is recovering.[10] Nurses often report that they "dislike" terminal patients and give them less attention in situations like Mrs. Morgan's floor where most of their work is routine and very monotonous. A significant number of the dying patients had illness problems that were personally repugnant: they smelled bad; they could not retain control of their bowels; they were in some cases disfigured from cancer, and so on. At the same time, while exasperated and irritated at the amount of time they had to give to terminally-ill people, nurses on Mrs. Morgan's floor had guilty feelings about the way the hospital and they themselves were failing these patients. The nurses had to listen to all the gripes and complaints of patients and families when physicians were neglectful and then were expected to control their own feelings and tongues when they would have liked to criticize the physicians and/or other nurses.

As with physicians, however, the underlying problem is the individual nurse's attitude toward death and dying.[11] When asked to comment on today's training of young nurses, an executive of a Visiting Nurse Association said: "Today's nurse is receiving more psychological preparation on terminal illness and is more sensitive to family needs. There is, however, no substitute for experience with dying persons, as well as for the maturity which comes from months and years of dealing in practical ways with the persons and concepts only discussed in school. Nurses who have been graduated in the last five years have received more specific preparation in the clinical care of the terminally ill. Perhaps this training is not adequate in all places, but nurses are far ahead of other health-care professionals in my judgment, in their skill and concern and in their attitudes when dealing with dying persons. Of course there are some insensitive and incompetent nurses, as there are physicians, but in these days, when nurses are struggling for more status and recognition of their professional expertise and skills, it is apparent that it is always difficult and often impossible for the nurse to function adequately in caring for terminally-ill persons, and many others, within the present structure of the health-care institutional system. Nurses must accept responsibility for making nursing-care decisions without first obtaining permission from a doctor, which requires that the nurse stay on the same case as hopefully the M.D. does. She must not be shifted away from the care of the person whose needs she has just begun to understand sufficiently to be able to make intelligent and informed decisions. For example, while it is the physician who signs the papers to allow a terminally-ill patient to go home, it is the nurse who has the planning responsibility, who instructs the family and patient on self-care at home. It is a nurse who visits the home to continue helping, supervising, and instructing the family and patient. Yet the rules of some of the best hospitals, such as Yale-New Haven Hospital, have not permitted the floor nurse, who has become the expert in many dimensions of a patient's problems, to visit patients at home after they leave the hospital—at least the nurse cannot be paid for such a visit. Many of course go on their own time, for which they receive no recognition or appreciation, except from the patient and family." [12]

Then what is the nurse to do, facing the "imperialism of physicians," when she discovers doctors who are lax in supervision or who are giving improper medication, or who are using terminally-ill patients for medical research and experimentation in improper ways? Also, there are nurses who have helped a cancer patient in terrible pain to die. "Sometimes," a nurse said, "the burden of decision of what to do is unbearable, more than anything else." Another nurse said: "One does not, in fact, agonize over the really difficult decisions or give adequate time to a patient like Mrs. Morgan because one is so busy with mundane chores. I need help, for example, in getting a patient's family off my back. I need help getting some of the physicians off my back, especially those who treat me like a machine. How am I supposed to treat Mrs. Morgan like a human being when the system doesn't treat me like one?"

Nurses who are better trained, with professional skills that deserve equal respect from other health-care persons, require a partnership or team relationship where collaboration, respect, mutual consultation and joint work is truly possible. Much lip service is given to teamwork in medicine, but the hospice movement is worth examining as the one place where there is effective teamwork which may well shed light on many other situations. An increasing number of highly trained nurses insist that they are colleagues to be consulted, not servants to be ordered around by doctors. Often, as nurses tend patients they become better informed of the current needs and situation of a specific patient than is the physician. Especially in the care of terminally-ill persons, the attending nurse knows far more of what is needed than does a non-hospital physician who simply drops by once in a while to look in and leave some instructions that the nurse may feel are ill-informed. Certainly a great deal of the new concern about more adequate care for dying persons has grown out of the observations of nurses; in fact, the attention to the hospice movement in England which has stirred new interest in more adequate terminal care in the United States reflects the extensive treatment of the subject in nursing journals.

Changing the System

Perhaps the only way to change a powerful, entrenched, effective health-care system is to confront it, from outside and within, with a counter-system that can demonstrate the need and possibility of change. Certain it is, that telling the story of one or two patients like Mrs. Morgan can have little impact beyond the immediate result of raising some questions and suggesting the need for more and deeper study of the situation. Mrs. Morgan's experience, however, is in striking ways parallel to other cases more thoroughly studied, such as in the case study of a dying woman called Mrs. Able and reported by Strauss and Glaser,[13] who examined the reactions of hospital staff and others in their book titled *Anguish*. Like Mrs. Morgan, Mrs. Able had a miserable experience in the hospital. She spent much of her time in tears and complaints, so that the hospital staff increasingly avoided her. The nurses did not so much deliberately neglect Mrs. Able, whose behavior they found to be disagreeable. It was just that the system simply led them to become less personal, more formal, more efficient in their routines of changing beds, feeding, giving medication. From Mrs. Able's perspective, however, the system failed in the first place because of the way different physicians and nurses gave her conflicting information, reflecting not only poor communication with her, but an obvious failure of team-work with each other.

The system also failed Mrs. Able, as it did Mrs. Morgan, because the nurses' solution was to send her home from the hospital to get her off their hands—even as at the same time they refused to let her keep control over her own life as she wished to do in the hospital. She was competent to give herself her own medication. Indeed, Mrs. Able kept careful records of what she was told, of what her medication was to be and when it was given to her. She was able to document the fact that she was neglected and could prove that she was not given adequate medication for her serious cancer pain. Perhaps because they had a bad conscience about the way the system treated Mrs. Able, the nurses rarely discussed her care and case with one another, and even refused to participate in a team conference which the chaplain wanted to set up to discuss Mrs. Able's case. So the system refused on the one hand to permit Mrs. Able to take charge of her own life, instructing her to take care of herself, give herself her own medicine, and so on; yet, on the other hand, the system also neglected her seriously instead of improving that care. Mrs. Able's physician tried to turn her over to the care of another doctor and he showed up rarely, often only at night when she was asleep. No one undertook to prepare her psychologically for her death.

Strauss and Glaser concluded that Mrs. Able could have been given a happier life in the hospital, "a considerably more compatible hospital career," if doctors and nurses had been trained to understand dying persons and their needs. Such training, they suggest, would focus on social relationships and teamwork. If the hospital staff was to accept responsibility for her quality of life until she died, the present system itself must be challenged at its center—that is, in the attitudes communicated in medical schools and training hospitals. Although teamwork is perhaps more advanced within medicine than in any other area of American life—much of the exceptional quality of performance and success in contemporary health care is the result of teamwork in practice and research—research into the experience of terminally-ill persons reveals a lamentable lack of communication, a serious deficiency in teamwork on the part of various health-care professionals. Further, if the medical profession is to work more effectively with dying persons, health-care professionals need partnership and more teamwork with members of related service professions, such as clergy and social workers. The hospice movement is one of the places where collaboration is being seriously developed and studied.

Mrs. Able's dying, Strauss and Glaser conclude, would have been much less stressful had the nurses been better informed and more understanding. But the institutional structures of the hospital and the health-care system seemed to prevent rather than to facilitate the needed sharing of information as well as discouraging cooperation among physicians, nurses, and others. Physicians and nurses, Strauss and Glaser concluded, need a better sociological-psychological orientation in the experience of dying persons before and after such patients enter a hospital, so that they can see the patients' need for more than impersonal medical treatment. Dying is, in any case, not the same for everyone. Each person's feelings about death are different, and in all cases the dying patient has a much greater need for human relationships and for counseling support than do other persons, and this is generally at a time when the patient is likely to be more and more isolated from the persons who might fulfill such needs. The system, however, provides no rewards or recognition for compassion, and the system of financial reimbursement gives no recognition at all to the needs of a dying patient for help other than strictly medical assistance. Rather than changing the system to equip and enable all health-care professionals to deal with dying persons—wherever they meet or find them—with more skill and compassion, the system, which relies on a depersonalizing sort of specialization, may be tempted to develop a new type of specialist: the physician who is called in just to handle dying persons. But Mrs. Morgan already had said that she felt like a machine on an assembly line, each new specialist pausing a moment to do his thing as she was moved on to the next, none of them knowing her and caring for her as a person.

The Environment for Dying

Earlier it was pointed out that the crucial element in the environment of terminally-ill persons consists of caring human beings and their attitudes, yet many people who labor to improve the environment of dying persons are too much concerned with architecture, furnishings, paint color, and medical efficiency. All of which suggests that for a variety of reasons institutions and professions fall far short of being and doing what they should be and do—a major problem being the failure of the imagination. The medical profession, which has worked miracles in dealing with the body, is slipping far behind in the realm of the spirit at the very time when the psychological factors involved in a cure are being rediscovered. For example, the desire to live is so crucial to a patient's success in a battle to save his or her life. Even in the most seriously ill cancer patients it is observed that a "lust for life" can make a tremendous difference. Yet that desire to live, which Mrs. Morgan had very strongly, was dissipated and perhaps even totally and needlessly destroyed by the health-care system itself, especially by the environment, which consisted essentially of human beings and their attitudes.

Mrs. Morgan said near the end of her life that it seemed

each time she succeeded in a resolve to "get hold of herself," she was set off again by the complaints of nurses and aides. Some of them would complain to her as if she could do something about hospital policy, and others sometimes came to a shouting match in the hall when she was trying to sleep, as they argued who was at fault when something was not done right. It was, she said, almost as if they were trying to tell her that she wasn't the only one who had problems. No doubt the environment of Mrs. Morgan's Intensive Care Ward was efficient and effective in all ways, except psychologically, its administrators and planners evidently had forgotten that social life, personal relationships, and the psychic environment may in the end be the most important aspects of human existence, even when it comes to prolonging life. Mrs. Morgan once asked, in a wry moment, why all the patients in the terminal-care ward weren't simply kept permanently under anesthesia. She knew nothing of the British hospice movement's insight that terminally-ill people can live to the end in environments that are joyously full of life and people. A physician who visited a British hospice described it as having a "remarkably peaceful and—dare I say it—distinctly joyful atmosphere," quite different from the grim workhouse environment where so many people like Mrs. Morgan groan away their last unhappy hours. The hospice helps the patient live in the present or the past, as desired, in contrast to the future orientation of the hospital where everyone lives to get out. The hospice, while stressing the importance of first-rate physical care and medical attention, is still able to see that for persons whose bodies are ebbing inevitably away, health for their remaining days must be defined in psychic terms, with new rituals developed to replace the typical hospital routines.

These new rituals, at their founding, must be personal, grounded in the individual wishes and needs of each patient. Instead of the tasteless semipopular music which flooded Mrs. Morgan's hospital ward, Mrs. Green's husband was able to have his records and tapes of music of his own choice, with both the time of playing and the selection under his own control. When Mrs. Morgan's daughter asked why her mother could not have some of her personal possessions in the hospital, she was told that it could not be permitted because there was so much theft in the hospital. Even an extra pair of stockings in a patient's drawer was almost certain to disappear. The hospital administration, therefore, was not willing to assume responsibility for anything the patient *valued*, even though it was precisely the souvenirs most valued that dying persons wanted to have with them. It is indeed ironic that western society cannot seem to provide safety and security for its elderly and sick, even in hospitals where they are dying. Still, when the focus shifts from warehousing the terminally ill, from custodial care to creating a nurturing and happy environment for them to enable their lives to find fulfillment and meaning at the end instead of a prolongation of misery, the human imagination can be stimulated to move in new and happy directions.

Since a high percentage of the terminally ill in the context herein described are cancer patients, and since cancer sometimes surprises everyone by reversing itself unexpectedly, some researchers suspect that the environment of the cancer patient should be re-examined. Terry, for example, says it is important to recognize that "the disease we call cancer is determined more and more by the ever-changing active states of the individual host who harbors the tumor, than by the history of cancer cells. It should be re-emphasized that the *ever-changing external environment* of the host plays a main role in the promotion or prevention of the development of a neoplasm." [14] Therefore, says Barbara Stewart, as long as one must pay attention to the wholeness and harmony of the individual and his or her environment, we should try to direct the energy of cancer patients toward alternatives for healthy re-patterning, for reawakening the human potention for self-cure. [15] She warns against dichotomies of "cause and effect, and internal and external," suggesting instead a focus upon "the patterning of disease that often evolves from the flow of energy between person and environment that is disharmonious with the life-process of well-being." Stewart quotes Goethe: "If we treat people as if they are what they ought to be, we help them to become what they are capable of becoming." [16] So, Stewart says, whether the patient lives or dies an effort should be made to enhance the full potential of life's being and becoming. There is no magic pill, just the possibility of repatterning the life situation of a patient so as to restore the balance of health and to harmonize the flow of energy through a life of quality, consistent with the process of well-being. The families Stewart works with support her assumption that patterning of ill-health evolves from an imbalance in the life situation of the patient, the illness not only accentuated by having to leave one's home and bed for a strange and miserable hospital environment, but also the illness may be stimulated and aggravated by family unhappiness or discord—that is, by a psychic environment that nourishes the disease instead of nourishing the patient. But Mrs. Morgan was victimized by a health-care system which increasingly seems to be more concerned with the disease than the person. How can such a mighty establishment be challenged?

FOR FURTHER READING

Abram, Ruth. *Not Alone with Cancer*. Springfield, Ill.: Charles C Thomas, 1974; Bernardi, R. and Hall, M. A., "Death in a Small Community Hospital," *Journal of the Kentucky Medical Association*, October 1969; Cramond, W. A., "The Psychological Care of Patients with Terminal Illness," *Nursing Times*, March 15, 1973; Duff, R. S. and Hollingshead, A. B. *Sickness and Society*. New York: Harper and Row, 1968; Holford, K. M., "Terminal Care," *Nursing Times*, Jan. 17, 1975; Stephens, Simon. *Death Comes Home*. Wilton, Conn.: Morehouse-Barlow Co., 1973.

4

The Hospice Concept in England

Searching for a model which might be adapted to the American scene to provide more human care for terminally-ill persons and to provide a basis for challenging the ingrained attitudes of the health-care establishment, a stream of American visitors—hospital chaplains, nurses, physicians, and others —began to arrive at British hospices in the early 1970's. One of them was Florence Wald, who was dean of the Yale University School of Nursing. Another was the Rev. Edward Dobihal, chaplain of Yale-New Haven Hospital, who also taught pastoral care at Yale Divinity School. Both of them had observed the way family, friends, and pastors often had to stand by helplessly as a dying patient was subjected to futile and useless routines designed to facilitate cure. As a hospital chaplain, Dobihal was committed to excellence in medical care and nursing for the terminally ill, but he had come to realize that it was useless for him or any other clergyman, for that matter, to try to talk to the dying patient in a way that might relieve fears and anxieties without dealing with the social situation that was aggravating—or in many cases actually creating—the fears and anxieties. He saw that an effective pastoral ministry to dying persons in the hospital had to re-establish and sustain close relationships between dying persons and their families, which was often impossible because the terminally ill were captives to respirators or other machines. He discovered that most people did not fear death itself so much as they feared the isolation and loss of freedom, the pain and suffering caused by the hospital environment itself.

But could that environment really be changed? Chaplain Dobihal recalled how the church, in an earlier generation, had experimented with the establishment of schools for children at a time when learning was only for the elite, providing models for society to follow; and also how the church had earlier developed hospitals which had become models for society's care for the sick. So he went to England to study the hospice movement, having heard of its success with a happier environment for persons with chronic degenerative disease and a limited life span. His focus was not merely on helping people die, but on helping them *really live* to the end of their lives. Despite a growing interest in death and dying, Americans, he found, still wanted to turn their eyes aside and shunt the terminally ill off into a corner where they could be ignored and forgotten. In such a situation he found it useless to talk or preach about anxiety unless he could help create some new "demonstration models" to show more constructive possibilities that would focus on a new kind of expertise which would make patient and family as comfortable and happy as possible, and which would allow both patient and family to participate actively in care and in fundamental decisions about the patient's life-style and treatment.

Dobihal was aware of the dangers involved in the word *model*, for in popular language the word is too frequently used for something to be copied. The hasty and sloppy way to seek to solve a problem is for community leaders to borrow blueprints from another community so they can construct a duplicate of the sort of program which apparently worked in the other community, forgetting or overlooking the fact that each and every community is unique, with its own varying needs, laws, and possibilities. A *model*, therefore, especially when the word is applied to a social institution or program, is primarily useful to stimulate the imagination and to define and open up the discussion to various alternatives and possible solutions to a problem, with the expectation that the blueprints for a recommended program in a specific community will vary considerably from the model developed elsewhere. For example, British law and funding procedures for institutions caring for the terminally ill were found by Wald and Dobihal to be quite different at many crucial points from those commonly available in the United States. British tradition, as reflected in the point of view and style of work in medical and social agencies, also varied. But they and other visitors to British hospices for the dying did find a challenging model: a style of institution, a program for pain care, an interdisciplinary team approach, and a point of view—all of which were needed and were adaptable to the American scene.

History of the Concept

The hospice movement in England is well-established, having slowly evolved across a century of tested experience. The women of a Catholic order, the Sisters of Charity, originated the idea of hospices for the dying in Ireland where in the middle of the nineteenth century they often found terminally-ill infirm people living and dying alone; or, more often, they found them in rural homes where a dozen persons were living in a two-room hut, the family lacking the space, time, energy and/or skill to care for them properly. First at Dublin and then elsewhere, these Irish nuns provided clean places where dying persons could be brought for loving care.[1] From Ireland this work of the Sisters of Charity expanded to England, and, as the program grew in insight and numbers of persons served, its influence spread to Asia, Africa, to Australia—but without any impact in the United States until the 1960's.

The flowering of the hospice movement in England dates from legislation in recent decades which made money available for such programs from the national health funds, although other agencies such as the Marie Curie Foundation, which was concerned with the care of cancer patients, also played a role. With funds available from these sources for research and experimentation, and with an experienced staff who were able to develop theory and procedures on the basis of careful evaluation of successful work, the hospices of England—now over twenty-five of them—were able to demonstrate the possibility of a radically different environment for the terminally ill.

St. Christopher's Hospice, in a London suburb, which drew special attention from these American visitors, opened in 1967, and two years later the cautious beginning of a home-care program was instituted. When visitors ask how St. Christopher's began, they are told the story of the young Pole who was dying of cancer in a London hospital.[2] "There ought to be a better way to take care of people in your condition," a nurse said to him one day. When that cancer patient died he left his savings of over a thousand dollars to begin a fund to start a hospice for the terminally ill. He had said to that nurse: "I will be your window in such a building." A staff member of St. Christopher's added: "With that as a start, we had no choice but to go ahead and create a place where patients could be surrounded with a more pleasant life."

The Hospice as Place

First of all, visitors see St. Christopher's Hospice as a place, a new kind of hospital especially created for the terminally ill. It is perhaps only natural that in an age when everything is institutionalized, American visitors would be searching for an alternative institution. The first thing one feels when visiting St. Christopher's or St. Joseph's Hospice, is a visibly different environment. St. Christopher's, although in London, is located away from the noise and rush and can have a garden with trees. It is a light, airy place with large open space which creates an atmosphere of sharing and community between patients and staff. St. Joseph's Hospice has windows reaching almost to the floor, so that a patient in bed can see across the gardens and into a busy adjacent street. The patient is thus not cut off from the rush of everyday life, but is able to see the turmoil of traffic—even the fire engines of the city neighborhood, which may well have been the patient's home. The staff found that to put a patient in a window bed was one of the best cures for depression, along with providing a garden to which patients could be taken into the sunshine. To visitors who anticipate a "death-house environment" with "cachetic, narcoticized, bedridden, depressed patients," the use of glass in the hospice is striking.[3] A multiple-storied building (because land was expensive), St. Christopher's patients (quoted in the 1974–75 annual report of the London hospice) describe it in a variety of ways—as a kind of convalescent home which is more like a family or as a "kind of annex to a hsopital where you can get better slowly or have comfort to the end."

In the front hall there is a metal plaque in memory of a young cancer patient who left his bequest for a window, and playing in the garden—invited there as part of the therapy —one often finds children of various races and colors, cheering the patients with the sort of happy noise which is excluded from a hospital ward. The furniture seemed to have none of the metal, antiseptic quality that the visitor has come to associate with hospitals. The patients at St. Christopher's who are not in wheelchairs are in low, simple beds which are as mobile as wheelchairs. The hospice beds have a canvas back sling which enables the patient to sit up with semireclining support, and each patient is supplied with five huge pillows. Some of the "dying persons" were actively involved in a wide variety of activities: drama, films, family celebrations, and so on. For the environment of the hospice is created in part by a different set of rules from the sort one finds in a regular hospital. Every effort is made to help patients continue with the life-style they are accustomed to. Not only is smoking allowed, for example, but patients who are used to drinking are given their cocktails.

Hospice as People

Whatever the rules, the architecture or the lighting, the quality of life and care which patients experience at St. Christopher's Hospice is determined for the most part by the skill, experience, and attitudes of the staff. From the moment patients arrive, they find their dignity respected and their wishes attended to with "warmth, empathy, and delicacy." [4] Admission and other routines are unhurried and are made occasions for expressing personal concern. In addition to finding at the hospice an active community of persons, patients also find a home-like atmosphere with places for their personal possessions, and with family rooms for visiting and for activities. It is a place where nurses feel free to sit on the bed of a patient, and where children, including babies, can come and go as they wish. At first it almost seems as if the patient has arrived at a club, with busy persons enjoying themselves with crafts, reading, following sports or whatever hobby they may enjoy.

Joan Kron has described St. Christopher's Hospice through the eyes of an American architect who went there to get ideas for designing a hospice in the United States.[5] LoYi Chan, as he packed in December of 1975 for his two-week trip to London, reported his puzzlement over whether or not to take his favorite red tie. In Canton, China, where he was born, red meant happiness and the color was never worn at funerals. He feared that the tie might not be appropriate at a hospice for the dying, but finally he packed it. He also took his wife along for the first time on a business trip because he felt that he was going into a situation where his emotions would be involved and he wanted her along to share in the experience. As with many other first-time visitors to a hospice they hardly knew what to expect. Incidentally, the director of St. Christopher's has said that many people expect it to be a place with a bit of religious music being played in the background, a gloomy place. But LoYi Chan said: "I don't know why I was worried about the tie. It was so cheerful there." He and his wife found a different emotional climate than they had expected, and any anxiety they may have had on arrival was quickly overcome by their experience with Dr. Cicely Saunders, the 56-year-old physician who perhaps more than anyone else is responsible for the conception of the place. Admirers of Dr. Saunders feel that to some extent the hospice concept has made such a powerful impact on many people because of the unique background and vision of Dr. Saunders as a result of her special preparation as nurse, social worker, and physician. She is a missionary of sorts for the terminally ill, because of the unique authority which she has earned.

When Dr. Saunders went to medical school at the age of thirty-three, with the announced aim of looking into the problem of pain and the dying patient, she "started rewriting the modern deathbed scene" in ways which may change all of our lives and the way we die regardless of whether we ourselves ever get near to St. Christopher's or not.[6] Dr. Saunders' vision is a simple one: an institution which combines excellent medical care with humane concern for persons—an institution which she herself describes as "a family community, a caring place." She has succeeded in creating such a backup institution for persons whose families cannot care for them at home; an institution of which a Harvard psychologist who visited it said: "I'd like to die at St. Christopher's."[7]

Another observer has said: "There is always kindness at St. Christopher's. Even the man who delivers the morning papers knows each patient by name." The nurses generally work in pairs so that the changes in bed linen, the lifting and turning, and so forth, can be accomplished with the least possible discomfort to the patient; indeed, they are turned into opportunities for friendly conversation. At St. Christopher's, one observer reported that she never saw "last stand" measures used to prolong the dying process—no respirators or feeding tubes.[8] Instead, she saw much attention given to the small details that mean so much to a patient: back rubs, pleasant baths, favorite foods. Even the scrubwoman, the cook, and the hairdresser view themselves as part of the "caring team," alongside the occupational therapist, the chaplain, the social worker, and the volunteers. Most of the patients, too, were caught up in the team spirit, seeking to minister to each other's needs and concerns.

Even the actual event of death was seen at St. Christopher's as being managed in such a way as to sustain the dignity of the dying person, and to help other persons in the hospice overcome their own fear of death. In most cases curtains were not drawn until the patient was actually dead, which enabled other patients and their families to observe the absence of patient distress and pain. Such procedure also guaranteed that no person felt left alone or abandoned at the moment of death. Dr. Liegner reported that other patients were thus helped to accept their own death without fear or dread, and even children who had known the dying person were able to accept the death with calm and assurance.[9] There was sadness on the part of patient and family at the final parting, but instead of leaving the deathbed with regretful memories, the family which had been helped at St. Christopher's to involve themselves in the dying person's care had good feelings, including the satisfaction of seeing that everything was done as the patient wished it.

The Hospice as Pain Care

American visitors to St. Christopher's Hospice were especially impressed by the pain-free comfort of dying patients they found there. Chaplain Dobihal was himself especially sensitive to the problem of pain. He had personally ministered to terminally-ill persons unable to enjoy their last days with family and friends because of burning pain, and had noted a British physician's conclusion that at least a fifth of dying hospital patients are in severe pain *which could be relieved.*[10] Of fifteen hundred British hospice patients, 70 per cent arrived at the hospice in severe pain. The first objective of the staff is to control that pain immediately, so that life quality can again be possible. Dr. Saunders and her staff at St. Christophēr's Hospice are successful in doing this in nearly every case.

Why does the American general hospital not do more to free dying persons from unnecessary pain? In part because the staff are devoted to cure, and lack the expertise which has grown up around the British hospices on how to care for terminally-ill people once all hope of cure has been given up. In principle, the medical staff of hospitals is devoted to preserving life at all costs and often does not pause to give attention to a range of needs and problems that do not fall within the scope of cure. As a result, hospital physicians and nurses are often reluctant to increase the dosage of pain-killing drugs, for fear that the patient will become addicted to the narcotic or that the drugs will interfere with the process of cure. At the heart of the hospice concept is a view of pain control which runs counter to the way a general hospital nurse is taught —*i.e.*, to withhold pain medicine until the patient demands it—or the hospital procedure by which a patient is given pain medicine on a fixed routine of every four hours even though he or she may begin to suffer serious pain within three hours. The staff at St. Christopher's Hospice assume that once it is definite that a person is dying, then the comfort of the patient takes precedence. Instead of waiting until a patient is miserable with pain to give relief, instead of waiting for the patient to demand the medicine because of his or her suffering, the hospice staff anticipates pain and gives the drug before the pain occurs, so that the patient never experiences any serious pain at all.

In their quest for happy and comfortable patients, the

hospice staff has noted that there are different kinds of pain, and that fear and anticipation of pain can be as uncomfortable and as painful as the misery caused by the disease. Palliation, therefore, requires pain medicine *before pain begins* in order to free the patient from that pain which is anticipation and dread. Once the patient discovers that it is again possible to be relatively free from pain, he or she relaxes and the psychological causes of pain disappear. "Pain," said a physician with experience in the British hospice, "is physical, psychological, but also social and spiritual."[11] To deal with all these elements requires therapy and expert skill in pain care. The debilitating power and extent of the pain which some dying persons experience, the British hospice people feel, has evidently been overlooked by many persons responsible for the care of the terminally ill. In order to restore the possibility of dignity, meaning, and happiness to a patient's last days, the staff at St. Christopher's take each symptom seriously and treat it with care. The hospice philosophy moves away from the negative view—that the patient cannot be cured—to the positive view that the patient has problems, and that pain is the principal one which the staff can do something about. It is reassuring to be able to tell patients that in 50 per cent of cancer cases there is no serious pain, but it is even more reassuring to be able to demonstrate—in cases of persons who arrive at a British hospice with pain that is already at an agonizing point—that debilitating pain is not inescapable after all. St. Christopher's staff holds that it is important and reassuring to begin pain control early, while the pain is still mild.

The sort of pain which a hospice physician calls "total pain" is nearly always made up of four elements: physical pain, mental, social pain, and spiritual. When a patient becomes increasingly anxious that the pain is going to get worse, insomnia and depression take over to aggravate the pain. It is much more difficult, hospice physicians have discovered, to deal with pain once the patient has been permitted to become depressed. So to control the pain the physician must deal with all four of its components, with the essential focus upon narcotics, because they are always needed. In the British hospices drugs are for the most part given orally in liquid form—rather than as injections or pills—in what is called Brompton's mixture or a Brompton cocktail. The liquid form makes it easy to increase or decrease the amount of drugs very slightly in order to adjust it precisely to the needs of a specific patient—in contrast to fixed-dose pills which are much more difficult to use in flexible ways. Brompton's mixture now generally includes fruit syrup, morphine and chloroform water, et cetera—a blend of ingredients based upon a hundred years of experience in England. Instead of administering pain-killing drugs of a fixed quantity, the hospice staff adjusts the dosage to whatever is required to control the patient's pain. What is important is the way the dose is administered during the day when the patient is awake, while at night the patient is able to sleep through until morning, a hypnotic may be added in the evening so that it will not be necessary to awaken the patient for a dose in the middle of the night. Not only is the frequency of administration adjusted to the need of a patient, but also the amount of narcotic. If a new patient arrives in agony, the hospice staff may initially administer a very large dose by injection. Then across the first three days the amount can be reduced gradually until the level of pain is discovered. The art of pain control, a British hospice physician suggests, is finding the gap which exists when the patient is not sedated. It may be very small, but it can be found if the liquid pain-control mixture is gradually reduced by very small amounts. Sometimes it is difficult to find that gap, but in a majority of cases the precise dosage can be found in this way; or the physician can work up to the proper dose level from a small dose at first which is gradually escalated until the pain is controlled—which may not require as much escalation as many persons might think, for patients reach a plateau which is often sustained for weeks or even months.[12]

Such pain control must be under the supervision of a

physician, which is perhaps why it is so often neglected in American nursing homes, where a doctor may visit only once a month. The art of giving the drugs to eliminate the pain before it becomes acute is comparable to the art of controlling diabetes, where the patient is given insulin in advance, to prevent a coma, rather than afterward to overcome it. For the first two or three days the hospice staff warns the patient that he or she may expect to experience sedation, but in a few days the effect is found to wear off with proper administration of the oral mixture, and the patient is then able to have a much more normal life-style than is usual in the hospital situation where a patient is given narcotics on a fixed schedule and dosage. Anxiety, depression, and psychological pain, the hospice staff has concluded, are compounded in many cases by typical hospital pain-control measures such as the administration of Demerol on a fixed schedule every four hours. The effect may last only two or three hours and the patient is frequently in serious pain before the schedule calls for another dose. So that psychological difficulties are compounded by the anticipation of the pain.

British procedures do not provide an exact model for American pain control, as the use of heroin is illegal in the United States. Alternative American procedures will be discussed in a later section, but, in general, the pain-control work of the British hospices has presented American medicine with an inescapable challenge. Perhaps the most important aspect of the challenge has been a tested answer to the worry of many physicians and nurses that serious addiction may result if a patient is given an adequate dosage of narcotics to keep him or her pain-free. On one hand, the British hospices challenge the danger philosophically, asking why addiction is an important factor in the case of a patient who is soon to die? The advantages of a comfortable and dignified life for the terminally-ill patient far outweigh any possibility of long-range addiction. On the other hand and even more important in this

British pain-control experience is the discovery that in a majority of cases drugs of addiction-level quantity are not needed for pain control, especially if psychological factors are skillfully handled from the beginning. In other words, if sufficient narcotic is used to eliminate pain completely from the very beginning, the patient is able to relax into freedom from anxiety. The discovery of the "gap," the precise level of pain, makes it possible to control a patient's pain with amounts of narcotic that fall below addiction levels, when the narcotic is not also needed to deal with pain caused by depression and other psychological factors resulting from periodic lapses in pain control.

A British hospice physician points out that giving drugs to people is not like feeding fuel into machines since each person responds differently to any one drug—which explains the few unusual cases where adequate pain control is not achieved through methods described in hospice procedures. *Each patient requires a particular tailor-made program of pain care*, not only in a continuing adjustment of the precise amounts of narcotic, but also in the combination of medication for other purposes. For example, the British hospice physicians recommend in some situations the use of steroids to stimulate the appetite and to contribute to the general sense of well-being, and sometimes to relieve painful inflammation around a cancer, and this despite possible side effects such as bloating, hair loss (which may have a psychological effect on a patient), or a perhaps 4 per cent increase in ulcers. Ulcers in terminal cases, like addiction, are less important than the improved life quality to be obtained if steroids help the patient recover strength or relieve breathlessness. In any case, a British hospice physician explains, each kind of pain has its own distinctive treatment and *the basic ingredient in most pain control is caring.*[13] A sensitive nurse or observer can tell if a patient is in pain simply by looking and listening: a wrinkled brow, tense hands, heavy breathing. But the nurse who is busy or the physician who assumes that the same fixed regimen of pain medicine can be mass-produced for all—and especially any persons, health-care professionals or not, who have never themselves suffered severe pain—may overlook such evidences of a patient's pain. And then say with cool objectivity, "That patient is always demanding attention, and one way is by complaining about pain."

Another worry of some physicians, when they initially examine this British hospice pain-control experience, is that because of an inhibiting effect on a patient's breathing or other consequences, larger doses of narcotics might shorten a patient's life. The British hospice, in theory, does begin with small amounts cf narcotic, gradually increasing the dosage to whatever amount is needed to control the pain. Dr. Lamerton, for example, feels that there need be no present maximum dose of pain-control medicine for a person who is dying.[14] The correct dose in his judgment may be five times what would normally be given if that is what a patient needs in such circumstances. But with constant pain control the amount of narcotics actually needed is much lower than physicians who have not worked with these procedures would expect. For example, where the usual starting dose of diamorphine (hesum) is 5 to 10 mg. given by mouth every four hours, only 13 per cent of patients are ever found to need as much as 30 mg., "which is a small quantity by any standard."[15] However, more importantly, instead of shortening the life of a patient who needs a very large dosage, patients actually may live longer, Lamerton says, because the narcotics—by relieving exhausting distress—enable the patient to get more rest, to eat better, and so on.

The British hospice physicians also recommend giving narcotics in a fluid mixture because this makes it possible to change the strength without changing the volume of dosage to deal with psychological factors which accentuate pain. Twycross points out that pain is a dual phenomenon consisting on one hand of the patient's perception of the sensation, and on the other hand of his or her emotional reaction to it.[16] Twycross also urges physicians to be alert to pain which is not physically based and which can best be treated by a "full and frank discussion." He tells of a cancer patient, for example, whose pain was not relieved by narcotic analgesics because it was the result of anger over the situation and the problems created by the unwillingness of doctors to discuss the case with her. Once this situation was dealt with, she no longer complained of pain.

Pain, of course, he points out, can also be aggravated by constipation, peptic ulcers, bedsores, hiccups, cystitis, muscle pains, and other conditions which require specific and immediate treatment, often by special nursing skills. Surgery may be required sometimes, simply to relieve symptoms which are preventing a dying patient from having a comfortable and happy life: to cut nerves, to open bowels, to drain fluids, or to reduce the pressure of large tumors, for example.[17] Vomiting, if not controlled by proper experimentation with anti-emetic drugs, may be due to a blockage which needs surgical attention. There are a variety of other irritations and symptoms which can be relieved promptly by medical personnel who are experienced in helping terminally-ill persons. For example, the British hospice physician suggests that honey with food will help relieve the unpleasant taste which is experienced by certain types of cancer patients.[18] As with serious pain, such things should be dealt with promptly, before they aggravate and contribute to psychological pain.

Since the aim of hospice pain control is life quality, to help a patient go home to live as long as he or she can with the assurance that acute pain need not be experienced again, pain relief in the hospice context also involves social and emotional support for the patient. Dr. Lamerton says: "Pain is not simply a matter of electrical impulses traveling up particular nerves, but is an expression of the way the whole individual meets the events of life." [19] Long-standing, relentless pain, he suggests, is almost a disease in itself because of the devastating effects it can have on a person. A patient cannot ever get away from it, so it commands the patient's attention while at the same time it seems to be a completely meaningless experience. As in a nightmare awful things seem to be happening to the patient, who fears that even more terrible things are about to happen in a milieu of terrible helplessness. Thus, exactly how and why a patient experiences pain may be complex and obscure, but it is colored with fear. Yet, the British hospice physician says, in most situations physicians and nurses do not tackle pain with sufficient confidence, and it is precisely in uncertainty that all kinds of terrors lurk for the patient. In the midst of such an experience it is essential, the hospice doctor feels, for the patient to have more than medication and good nursing, since social life and human relationships are the best antidote to fears and to emotions which may aggravate pain.

Dr. Twycross, formerly research specialist at St. Christopher's Hospice, and now medical director of a new hospice at Oxford, reports the discovery by a group of general practitioners that as the doctor-patient relationship improved, the dosage of drugs often could be reduced.[20] "This almost certainly," he said, "reflected the doctor's own feelings." Once the physician was able to deal with his own pain which resulted from the patient's dying, the needs of the patient for drugs became less. On the other hand, when a patient came to feel that the physician was not being totally honest or was trying to cheer him by saying: "You're coming along fine," the patient—increasingly retreating into himself, feeling alone, feeling more and more lonely and dejected—came to need more and more drug relief, a need intensified by his resentment and emotional pain. At the heart of the hospice concept, therefore, is an understanding of the need for pain control which challenges the entire health-care system at points more crucial than the type and amount of narcotics given.

For example, a London physician complained to a hospice

doctor that he was giving adequate narcotics to a patient every two hours and it was having no effect at all. The hospice staff member asked: "Have you sat down to talk with him?" The other physician said: "Have I what!" The hospice staff member persisted: "Sat down to talk with him! The mental anguish is quite as bad as the physical, and the drugs you are using are for acute pain, not this sort of chronic pain." [21]

Hospice as Point of View

One does not discuss pain care, nor any other aspect of the hospice approach to terminally-ill persons, except in the context of a total point of view which runs counter to much of what is currently dominant in the medical establishment. This is not necessarily a new point of view, of course, since it was long that of the small-town family doctor, and of the visiting nurse organizations which as long as seventy-five years ago were developing and living such views. Nor do persons in the hospice movement—even as questions are raised and institutional challenges are presented—intend to be negatively critical of medical personnel. Hospice leaders view themselves as working within the health-care system as an ongoing part of the continuing process of self-criticism and self-improvement which had led to so much excellence in medical research and care. The mention of small-town physicians and nurses of seventy-five years ago might serve to reinforce the prejudices of some who suspect that hospice people are saying that "tender loving care" is more important than medical science, or that "tlc" is all that is needed by the terminally ill. Nothing could be further from the truth. The hospice movement in Britain and elsewhere is firmly committed to excellence in medical care, to defending and justifying its point of view by scientific research in keeping with the best of current work in the health-care sciences. Indeed, far from advocating "tender loving care" instead of science, the hospice staffs are asking if in order to be more scientific and effective, medical care doesn't also need more "tender loving care." Conclusive research evidence demonstrates that far from being as scientific as they would aim to be, countless physicians and nurses have —perhaps unconsciously—held points of view which are not scientific at all, with regard to death and dying, but which have simply reflected the taboos and unexamined values of an often superstitious society.

Far from being critical, even at this point, the aim of the hospice movement is to provide collaborative support for health-care professionals, and indeed for all persons who are involved with the terminally ill, so that taboos can be replaced with tested skills and with expertise which is rooted not only in deeper experience but also in experimentation, testing and demonstration. The hospice point of view begins with the conviction that much more than "tender loving care" is needed, and that as with any other medical skill, the care of the dying is to be learned by practice and demonstration. For this reason hospices are needed, not only as places in which to care for the dying but also as teaching and training centers where medical students, nurses, and others can gain firsthand knowledge— and the proper point of view toward death, dying, and the care of the terminally ill. Some critics of the hospice movement have worried about implications of euthanasia, or at least a diminishing of aggressive life-prolonging therapy. Dr. Lamerton, however, points out that the euthanasia issue becomes much less important when terminally-ill persons are made happier, for they then have a greater desire to live. The desire to live is also closely related to personal relationships, and central to the hospice point of view is the conviction that the whole family must be treated, and not merely the patient in isolation. The hospice unit of care is the patient-and-family, for families have a role to play both in sickness and health. The need of persons to be responsible for each other and to take care of their own health needs becomes crucially relevant with dying persons, a community of friends and loved ones constituting the environment which is essential for the well-being, comfort and care of the terminally ill. Therefore the hospice point of view focuses upon freeing the family to be together, rather than increasing their separateness and burdens as is so frequently the case otherwise.

As seen in the discussion of pain care, the hospice point of view as it has emerged in Britain has sought to refocus medical care on a concern for the individual person's uniqueness. If the patient's spark of life is to be valued to the extent that the medical profession devotes heroic measures to prolong it, then the quality of that life is to be valued even more. Symptom control and spiritual support are therefore seen to be two essential and interrelated elements of care, with the total well-being and life-style of each patient seen as central. The goal of hospice care is to enable the patient to continue life as usual, enabling each person to continue work, family life, or whatever seems especially significant to him or her, enabling the patient to feel that one's last weeks are part of an ongoing life. The hospice point of view combines elements of life that have too long been separated in modern specialization, such as the pastoral and the medical. The hospice point of view is religious in that it affirms the value of personality and not merely physical existence. It is rooted in philosophical themes that value life and believe in sources of help which transcend the capacity of any one person or group to exist meaningfully alone.[22] Hospice approaches to care of the dying help them deal with emotions in healthy ways. Instead of saying about the wife of a terminally-ill man: "Wasn't it great that she had such self-control that she hardly cried at all?" the hospice staff member wants to say: "How wonderful that she could cry so freely." [23] But the significant thing, to the hospice staff, was that the wife of the dying man was able to remain with him to the very end. And despite her own sorrow, instead of feeling helpless and unable to do anything she could actively assist him in dying without feeling guilty of doing the wrong thing. She could hold his hand as a last channel of reassurance. She could see that—instead of distress or suffering as he died—her husband was able to withdraw into a rather beautiful giving-in to serenity, slipping away gently as a calm wave retreats into the ocean.[24] Thus the hospice concept, Dr. Lamerton suggests, is rooted in the gospel, St. Luke 2:29–31: "Lord, let thy servant depart in peace."

Such a point of view is possible at the British hospice because it is embodied concretely in what human staff members and family members are enabled to say and do. A point of view which does not close dying persons up in a dark place, but bathes them in sunlight and fresh air, which seems to pervade not only the architecture but also the attitudes of staff members such as the nurse who said that it was a privilege to be able to perform that last act of service of washing the dying patient, or the chaplain who said: "That dying woman enriched my life so much more than I was able to enrich hers." In a context where everyone seeks to receive as well as give, the hospice staff becomes a place of peace for families and health-care professionals as well as for patients.

The Hospice as Teamwork

If the environment is persons, it is enabled by teamwork of persons who accomplish more human care because of their willingness and skill in working together across interdisciplinary lines. Physicians and nurses are usually too busy to take the time necessary to resolve tensions between each other or to learn adequately from each other, much less with clergy, social workers and others. The hospice concept in England rests firmly on the assumption that every person who comes into contact with the dying person needs to be a member of the caring team—even dying patients themselves in nearby beds. Such persons, even the health-care professionals, have too often worked at cross purposes. In the hospice the staff meet regularly for detailed discussion of each patient and family, so that everyone is thoroughly informed and in agreement on procedures, and in more than words this collaboration and teamwork is reflected in every aspect of the care. Even the cleaning staff understand themselves to be partners—not merely in an important enterprise, but in personally giving loving care and attention to patients. Indeed, a specific patient may choose to discuss needs or problems with the hairdresser or cook, instead of the physician, and even among the health-care professionals individual prerogatives and overspecialized roles begin to crumble. The chaplain may find himself asked to rub a patient's back, and that same patient might ask a physician to pray. The social worker's theory about how a particular patient's disease is going to progress is heard in staff meetings alongside the physician's, who comes at the same time to see that some of the staff members, such as nurses who spend the most time with patients, may have the best insight into medical needs and procedures for meeting them. Basic questions of medical ethics also may be brought to the team's attention by lay volunteers.

Concern for human beings, in other words, comes to transcend roles and prerogatives so that teamwork comes to blend a variety of insights and skills into a new wholeness of purpose and possibility. Where the hospice experience of a patient like Mrs. Morgan was made miserable by the coming and going of impersonal specialists, none of whom seemed willing to answer her specific questions, the patient at the British hospice deals with a team of persons each of whom pauses to answer any question, and who support each other and co-ordinate their efforts closely to keep the needs of the dying person foremost in their attention. Teamwork has in many ways been more advanced within the medical system than in any other professional area, yet even in medicine it has been fraught with tensions, jealousies, conflicts, empire building, and disagreements on fact and principle—often at the expense of the patient. Medical science has in our time accomplished remarkable advances through teamwork in practice and research: ability to use the chemist's genius, the surgeon's knife, the therapist's imagination and skills. But the hospice concept challenges the health-care system to even more exciting developments as interdisciplinary teamwork is made more effective within, and is further extended to include more effective and significant co-operation with research and professionals outside, the field of medicine. It is not only at the time of death that a human being's needs are mental, emotional, and spiritual as well as physical, and each person needs to interrelate with others to replace, to nurture, the hope and love that can transcend pain and sickness.

A visitor to a British hospice may at one moment be shocked to discover that the weekly clinic for outpatients is turned into a social event with fun and refreshments . . . but why not? Teamwork and sharing not only enhance the capacity to be understanding of others, but also improve the ability of each team member in common-sense ways as well as in professional skills to become more adaptable and flexible in the ability to work with others. Not only are role definitions and job descriptions continually changing and growing, but so are the sort of personal relationships that enable people to help each other, support each other, even evaluate each other constructively and co-operatively. Being open and willing to talk in a team relationship creates a willingness to accept limitations and a need for help, makes it possible to share weaknesses as well as strength. New persons, or young persons in training, can not only learn skills through demonstration and observation but also can be transformed by a community which lives a point of view. On the basis of his experience with hospice teams, Dr. Lamerton points out that instead of trying to work separately, doctors and nurses develop the sort of team spirit which is desired elsewhere but is so often lacking.[25] Instead of dominating from their role as authority figure, physicians come to learn from and accept support as well as give support as each member of the team becomes "more alive, intelligent, and human"—physiotherapists, occupational therapists, social workers, laboratory technicians, and a variety of other skilled workers caught up in the emerging, co-ordinated whole.

Place of Life, Not Death

The spirit of St. Christopher's Hospice in London is in many ways the spirit of its imaginative founder and medical director, Dr. Cicely Saunders, who has helped communicate its insights regarding the sensitive handling of medical, emotional and spiritual needs of the terminally and chronically ill, and their relatives, to visitors from many continents. St. Christopher's Hospice has inpatient wards, an outpatient clinic, a home visiting service, a day-care center for children of staff members, and private accommodations for the elderly—combining all these elements into a remarkable environment. It has been suggested that life at St. Christopher's Hospice is illustrated by the variety of announcements to be found on its bulletin board.[26] At one time recently there were to be found on it the following: There was a diagram showing how mounting expenses for staff salaries, and so on, have been met by money from teaching hospitals, tax funds, and gifts from individuals. There was the announcement of the birth of a baby set alongside a list of anniversaries of patients who died in that week a year ago. There was a list of chapel announcements, of social and other less serious meetings, and a request for goldfish to restock the pond. Through all of this there is a spirit which values life, and affirms death not as something morbid, but as another of the events of human life which can be honored and valued along with birth and the other basic experiences. If it is a model, a challenge to the health-care system, it is not because the hospice set out to be those things, but simply because it set out to be a human place that does an important medical work with excellence.

FOR FURTHER READING

Other readings on British hospices: "Haven of Peace," *Nursing Times*, Vol. 69, no. 33, Aug. 16, 1973; Lamerton, R. C. "The Need for Hospices," *Nursing Times*, Jan. 23, 1975; Saunders, Cicely, "The Last Frontier," in Reaves, R. B. *et al.*, *Pastoral Care of the Dying and the Bereaved*. New York: Health Sciences Publishing Corp., 1973; Saunders, Cicely, "The Moment of Truth," in Bloom, *op. cit.*

Recommended readings on British pain-control methods and their evaluation: Evans, R. J. "Experience in a Pain Clinic," *Modern Medical Care*, 1971, 16 (10), p. 7; Jaffe, J., "Drug Addiction and Drug Abuse," in Goodman, L. S. *et al.*, *The Pharmacological Basis of Therapeutics*. New York: Macmillan Co., 1975; LeShan, L. "The World of the Patient in Severe Pain of Long Duration," *Journal of Chronic Dis.*, 1964, 17, p. 119; Marks, M. D. and Sachar, E. J., "Undertreatment of Medical In-patients with Narcotic Analgesics," *Am. Intern. Med.*, 1973, 78, p. 173; Mount, B. M. *et al.*, "Use of the Brompton Mixture in Treating the Chronic Pain of Malignant Diseases," *Canadian Medical Association Journal*, 1976, 115, 2, p. 122; Twycross, R. C. "Euphoriant Mixes," *British Medical Journal*, 1973, 3, pp. 552 ff; "Clinical Experience with Diamorphine in Advanced Malignant Disease," *Int. Journ. of Clinical Pharmacology*, 1974, 9, p. 189.

The New Haven Hospice:
An American Adaptation

The hospice concept has appeared on the North American continent in a variety of forms. The Catholic Order of the Hawthorne Dominicans has operated seven highly regarded nursing homes for the care of terminally-ill people, including one on the Lower East Side of New York City. Calvary Hospital in northern Manhattan, also a Roman Catholic institution, has provided terminal care for indigent dying persons, and is an able representative of specialized hospitals which accept referrals from public hospitals and Medicaid-supported nursing homes. Youville, a Catholic hospital in Cambridge, Mass., which has specialized in long-term rehabilitation and chronically-ill patients, has in recent years added a counseling program for dying persons in conjunction with the Boston Theological Institute. Some other hospitals, like Royal Victoria Hospital in Montreal and St. Luke's Hospital in New York City, are developing special "hospice" units within the walls and structure of the general hospital,—and so are other hospitals. But the Branford Hospice at New Haven, Conn., is perhaps the best known established effort to adapt the British hospice institution to the American scene.[1] It has been established to be an experimental model to serve the rest of the country in staff training, research, and demonstration. It therefore deserves close attention from those interested in improving the quality of care for our terminally ill.

Why New Haven? Other communities might have acted first to create a demonstration model, but a unique combination of factors spurred concerned persons around Yale University and the New Haven community to take advantage of resources available to make the experiment possible in that location. New Haven county has a population of nearly 750,000 people, with both urban and rural areas, with a sufficient number of terminally-ill persons to justify the existence of a hospice program. Near by are a Veterans Administration hospital with terminally-ill patients, the large teaching hospital related to Yale University Medical School, and a community-based hospital. Physicians, clergy, visiting nurses, the faculty of health-care training institutions in New Haven all had shown a growing concern for deficiencies in the care of terminally-ill persons in the community. In addition the city had often shown its willingness to serve as the place for experimental programs funded by private foundations or by the Federal government.

A catalyst, perhaps essential to move persons from concern to action, came in 1964. A new chaplain at Yale-New Haven Hospital spent his first year there learning and listening.[2] Noticing the difficulty chaplains had in ministering to dying persons in the hospital and to their familes, he was drawn to attend a 1966 symposium on death and dying conducted at Yale by Dr. Elisabeth Kübler-Ross. He thus became acquainted with the work of Dr. Cicely Saunders of St. Christopher's Hospice, who at that time was at Yale as a visiting professor at the School of Nursing. A number of key persons in New Haven were impressed by the graphic picture of human need which Dr. Kübler-Ross painted at the symposium. She noted that terminally-ill persons were often treated as having no rights or opinions of their own, and given no opportunity to share in decisions about their treatment and care. Indeed, she said, the dying person who tried to protest the continual X-rays, blood tests, electrocardiograms, infusions, transfusions, heart machines, and so on, might be sedated and made helpless in order to prevent further protests. A dying person may cry for peace and rest, may simply ask one person to delay treatment to answer one question, but instead "he will get a dozen people around the clock all busily preoccupied with his heart rate, pulse, electrocardiogram, or pulmonary functions, his secretions or excretions, but not with him as a human being." [3]

Reporting on the response of clergy, nurses, physicians, and others to that symposium, Chaplain Dobihal said: "Those 1966 speakers raised our consciousness, but we were a group of loners, with different kinds of feelings. Some of us were angry about the lack of care or the incompetence; others were confused about what they were supposed to be doing." Also as Dobihal and others continued to discuss the challenge and the needs they saw, it was difficult for any of them to get out of their role, to avoid speaking defensively as a nurse, a doctor, or a clergyman. It was only natural to try to place blame on others. A concerned group of persons, however, continued to meet regularly, conscious of the challenge of Dr. Kübler-Ross that they should try to listen to terminally-ill persons themselves as human beings with a right to be heard and as persons whose dying experience could be of help to many other persons, if properly understood. The group meeting in New Haven were also moved by the statement of Dr. Saunders that at the heart of the problem of the terminally ill was a failure of teamwork—especially a failure of physicians, social workers, nurses, clergy, pharmacologists and others to cross interdisciplinary lines to meet human need.

Dobihal himself, because of a recurring physical ailment of his own, knew how debilitating pain could be and how hard it was to be human before the pain was reduced. Further, as he sought to design and define his hospital ministry he became convinced that neither he nor any other clergyman could adequately minister to a dying person and the family without helping them resolve the conditions which caused so many of their fears and anxieties. He felt intuitively that a religious atmosphere of caring, love, concern, and understanding was central to a ministry to dying persons, but he also was convinced that authentic religion had a prophetic aspect. The church, for example, could not adequately minister to black persons who were victims of anxiety-producing prejudice without undertaking the prophetic task of working for justice for them. And the prophetic task in relation to the all too prevalent prejudice against dying persons, which he saw in the vision of Dr. Cicely Saunders, lay in facilitating a new model for terminal care which might demonstrate new alternatives. He therefore took a sabbatical year from his work in 1970–71 in order to go to England to study the hospice concept.

Initial Exploration

The exploratory group which had grown out of the Kübler-Ross symposium in New Haven had by 1967–68 identified a group of neglected patients and had begun the process of defining the nature of the problem and the needs to be served by a new approach to the terminally ill. The group pursued an interdisciplinary approach, consulting with various hospitals and agencies, carefully informing themselves of what was actually going on and what might be possible. Some members of the group were motivated by intensely personal concerns. A pediatrician was concerned with problems created for some of his child patients when they were ignored or were not informed and involved when a family member died. Another physician in the group was irritated at the poor care his mother was getting in a nursing home and the way he was shoved aside by the bureaucracy of the institution. Some members of the group were visionary, some were more practical and realistic, but as they consulted with specialists on pain control, for example, it became clear to them that the different professionals involved with the terminally ill could work together more effectively for the good of the patient, and could and should take more of a team approach in which they would be more supportive of each other.

These conversations and explorations gradually matured into the conviction that they should take initiative to form a new and separate institution for the care of terminally-ill persons, an institution outside of and supplementing existing facilities, agencies, and programs of the health-care system. One aim was to challenge and if possible influence the entire system. Although the importance of home care for dying persons was in their thinking from the beginning—mounting hospital costs were already causing many persons in the medical establishment to give thought to home care for all sick persons —the New Haven group assumed that it should make the effort involved in adapting and building upon the British hospice model as the best available experience they could test and modify. Since they were setting out to establish a new type of institution for the New Haven region, they faced a continuing struggle, especially with the press, to avoid having the hospice program labeled as just another kind of hospital, a special facility for dying persons. A hospice facility was needed, they felt, for dying persons who had no home, for others whose families had quarters so cramped or inadequate that proper care would be difficult or well-nigh impossible at home, and for many others for various reasons—enough to justify a construction program. But in the drive for funds, planning with contractors and architects, and all that goes with building, it was soon seen as essential that the construction aspect should not become the "tail that might wag the dog."

Beginning Organization

The structure of an organization can also lead groups astray from their central vision and primary aims. It was, therefore, important to draw many other community leaders, especially those essential for organization, into the vision and study. A hundred and fifty persons thus became involved in task forces on community relationships, finance, building and site, and so on. Volunteers assembled the data required to request "seed money" to employ some staff from foundations. The chairman of the board said: "The task forces were important in building community consciousness and support. It was easy to assume that we had more support than we had, that more people understood the need than actually did, and that influential leaders would jump on our bandwagon once we started to roll. In fact, however, we had to define the gap in the health-care system to sell our program as an experiment worth trying. . . . In other words we were involved in criticizing the system, which naturally caused some resistance, with health-care people asking: 'Why can't we do this through our present institutions and programs?' "

The initial steering committee included a woman doctor whose husband was a Yale chaplain; a pediatrician who taught at Yale Medical School, along with a professor of clinical surgery from the same faculty; many of the most interested persons were nurses, however, some whose consciousness had been raised by the teaching and presence of Dr. Cicely Saunders during the year she was at Yale Nursing School. Florence Wald, dean of that school from 1958 to 1967, and who later became Coordinator of Inpatient Planning for the New Haven Hospice, played a crucial role in stirring up interest in the idea. She was principal investigator in two studies of care for dying patients under grants from the United States Public Health Service and the American Nursing Foundation. As a result of these studies, a report, "An Interdisciplinary Study of Care for Dying Persons and Their Families," was prepared with the collaboration of Chaplain Dobihal, Dr. Morris Wessel and Dr. Ira Goldenberg, both of whom continued to play key roles in the hospice structure.

Upon the foundation of such work and study it was possible to conduct a research conference in October of 1970, and to create the task forces in May of 1971; then, in November of 1971, the New Haven Hospice was incorporated as a non-profit corporation under Connecticut law. By March of 1972 the formal organization of the board of directors, with Chaplain Dobihal as chairman, was completed. Florence Wald and her husband, who also served on the hospice board, visited St. Christopher's Hospice five times between 1967 and 1975—this being another part of the contribution which such members of the initial group made to the task forces on patient care, professional relations, internal organization, research, and so on.

Finding the Right Staff

The New Haven observers of British hospice programs saw that the most important part in their success was finding the right staff persons, a procedure much more important and crucial than any other single item in making possible a program and environment which could accomplish the objectives and sustain the hospice point of view. In the British hospices it was not necessarily the person with the largest salary, the greatest amount of education, or the most imposing title, who was crucially helpful to a specific patient. The woman who did the laundry, for example, had a special touch and relationship with persons as she went from bed to bed, and the cockney housekeeper had a special impact upon persons with her sort of background. But however important all these persons might be, there could be no hospice program until there was a physician on the staff who was a specialist in pain control and in other dimensions of work with the terminally ill, and until a director of nursing could be found who was committed to the hospice concept. Finding such a physician is a difficult task. As one young physician said, speaking frankly, "There isn't much money and future in working with the dying." And a young surgeon who served as a member of a hospice team said: "Other physicians sometimes say that they admire my dedication and sense of purpose in being willing to do this, but I must admit to worrying once in a while about what they really think. Do they see this work as a foolish detour which can only handicap my career as a surgeon?" Another physician in a similar position said: "I'm not really worried about the effect on my long-range career of a period of time serving on a hospice team, because I am firmly convinced that the hospice concept is going to spread throughout the entire health-care system, so that in twenty years it will be taken for granted as being as essential as cardiac units are now. But certainly there is the risk that some patient or family member who knows of my identification and reputation with the terminally ill may panic and assume things that are not so when they learn I am to perform surgery." A physician who served on a committee to look for a medical director for a hospice said: "Not only are we running counter to attitudes taught and reinforced in the teaching hospitals—that doctors should be concerned only with cure, not palliation—but even young physicians who become interested in our vision and goals are warned by colleagues and medical school teachers: 'Don't do it! You don't want to be labeled as a death specialist. You may never live it down!' "

In any case, few American physicians had the expertise developed at the British hospices, so in 1973 when Dr. Cicely Saunders came again to New Haven, she showed a film on her hospice program in England to nearly a thousand persons,— the number attending was an indication of the extent to which interest in the idea had grown in the New Haven community.

In the course of showing the film, she said: "You need a specialist for the development of your hospice program in New Haven, so I suggest that you give careful attention—as you watch this portion of the film—to the work of Dr. Sylvia Lack, who is shown here interviewing at St. Christopher's Hospice." As a result of this film introduction, Dr. Lack was invited to New Haven and was employed as medical director of the New Haven Hospice, thus bringing to America her own expertise as well as information and experience she could share from her work at St. Joseph's and St. Christopher's Hospices in England. Dr. Lack also served in New Haven with a joint teaching appointment in the Department of Internal Medicine at Yale University School of Medicine.

Through a similar referral process, New Haven Hospice was able to secure the services of Sister Mary Kaye Dunn as director of nursing. Sister Mary Kaye was working as head nurse on a medical floor, dealing with advanced cancer patients at St. Mary's Hospital which is affiliated with the Mayo Clinic at Rochester, Minnesota. As Clinical Nursing Consultant to hematologists and hematologic oncologists there she became increasingly dissatisfied with the way she saw dying persons scattered over the hospital. She wished to equip herself to work more effectively with dying persons, so she consulted Dr. Kübler-Ross about the possibility of going to England for a visit to St. Christopher's Hospice. Instead, Sister Mary Kaye came to New Haven where she could be involved in the learning experience of a new institution where everything was open for experimentation and investigation. When she and Dr. Lack arrived in New Haven in September of 1973, they found that a great deal of advance thinking and planning had taken place, but they were faced with two tremendously difficult tasks:

—to develop a team, which would begin by learning to work with one another and then with others;

—to develop the hospice program from scratch.

As the chairman of the hospice board admitted to them:

"Our idealism has not yet been spelled out adequately in concrete ways." Dr. Lack and Sister Mary Kaye found plenty of support, but faced much hard work. One of them later said: "I would not advise another hospice project to bring two new patient-care people from out of town to develop their own job descriptions and program, including such matters as interagency agreements, legal questions, procedures, insurance, reimbursement financing, and other matters which require more skill and background in administration and planning than a physician and nurse are likely to have."

Still, though its efforts to recruit public health nurses who were prepared and experienced in home care had not been successful, the hospice board of directors was able to move ahead with staff who were committed to the hospice philosophy. Dr. Lack and Sister Mary Kaye began by going camping together to get better acquainted and talking plans through late into the night until they knew where to begin and what to do. In December of 1973, Dennis Rezendes, an experienced administrator who was well acquainted with the business and political structure of the New Haven community came to the staff, and by 1975 there was a staff of twenty-two full and part-time employees, including a director of research and a director of volunteers, as well as nurses, office workers, and many others. The hospice began with a board of directors of nine persons. As the chairman explained: "Since we had all suffered within hierarchical systems, we didn't want a chief. We tried to work democratically, even when we later expanded the board to nineteen so as to include persons with skills in fundraising and administration. I have a concept of organization as needed to accomplish a task, but also as a help in getting our primitive anxieties under control. This thought, too, came from England, from the Tavistock philosophy that every organization has its support function for the sickness that exists in an organization."[4]

A major issue was selecting an administrator for the health-care organization. Said another member of the hospice board, "One problem with having a boss . . . results from the tendency of everyone to defer to physicians, and from the expectation of doctors that the pecking order will operate to their advantage. If the executive is a physician, then nurses and others in the organization may be psychologically subjected to domination as they are on the hospital floor. On the other hand, if the executive is not a physician, teamwork and democracy may be equally frustrated, as the executive finds that there are competitive underground power bases which he, as a non-medical person, is unable to control or handle. Many hospitals and agencies try to solve this dilemma by employing executives who are neither physicians nor nurses but who have special training in the language of medicine and in administration. We could, for example, have hired someone trained in hospital administration. But no amount of care in staff selection can avoid role conflict among board members and staff members in a program where dynamic and creative persons are called together to create something new, especially when some of these individuals are busy physicians accustomed to decision-making, and to division into specializations wherein each person defers to others in their areas of authority. The hospice concept seeks from the beginning to blur role difference and to question authority procedures in order to establish new approaches to teamwork."

The New Haven hospice staff and volunteer leaders approached their new tasks with optimism of the sort described by Seymour Sarasen who has studied the intentions and efforts of new agencies to change radically the styles of work and structures which they impatiently endured in other social agencies they had found to be ineffectual.[5] Despite an awareness of Sarasen's research showing how the old habits and patterns of organization inevitably creep in to shape the future of a new structure in ways contrary to the organizers' intentions, even before the organizers are aware of them, members of the hospice board and staff have had to deal with serious conflict, even with the discovery that some people find it impossible to continue working together no matter how idealistic and well-intentioned they are. In a situation of inevitable role conflict and fatigue, therefore, a successful interdisciplinary team requires serious attention to team-enabling, perhaps with one person assigned to the task of monitoring team functioning. And because of the heavy emotional load of dealing continually with death and grief, the staff of a hospice—more perhaps than any other agency—has found it essential to have a staff psychiatrist to provide continuing support for the staff and to help keep teamwork alive.

New Haven Hospice as Organization

The best ideas soon wither and die unless they attain institutional shape and financial support—which requires almost interminably tedious hard work by human beings. Hospitals themselves illustrate how, even then, such institutions tend to become self-serving, with the persons who had the vision to initiate the institution finding themselves in a back seat as employed professional staff develop their own views and fight for preferred methods of work. While the supportive organization of New Haven Hospice actually began with the employment of a planning and development staff, the crucial importance of the Medical Advisory Committee and National Advisory Committee of twenty-four prominent people should not be overlooked, for the hospice's goal of serving as a model to influence similar developments across the country required a continuing research effort. It may well be that a strong emphasis on research is essential if Federal government funding is to be secured, since members of grant committees at the National Cancer Institute and elsewhere are likely to be research oriented. Raising money from foundations, as well as from individuals in the community, also requires a base of careful research, advance planning, well-defined conceptual goals, slow and thorough consultation, careful preparation of legal permissions, and public relations efforts. All this requires money. New Haven Hospice has been able to demonstrate excellence in its pilot program because of a fifteen-month grant from the National Cancer Institute in the autumn of 1974, later renewed until the fall of 1977. Funds were also secured from the Van Amerigen Foundation, the Sachem Fund, and other sources. This enabled the hospice board and staff to describe itself as "a nonprofit, tax-exempt corporation in the state of Connecticut involving health professionals and community representatives who have organized to plan, design, and implement a community program for the terminally ill," and to publicize their program as the "first and only comprehensive program for the terminally ill and their families in America." Later they added: "The hospice staff is the most unique assemblage of talent and experience in dealing with the terminally ill now available in America."

Establishing a new structure and facility involved a great deal of hard work. In August of 1973, endorsement was received from the Connecticut State Council on Hospitals for a 44-bed chronic disease hospital, with the condition: sixty days to find a site in New Haven, Seymour or Ansonia. Finding a proper site in one of the approved locations turned out to be impossible within that amount of time because of opposition of the residents who misunderstood the hospice concept, imagining the facility as a gloomy place from whence dying people might wander outside to molest neighborhood children.

In May of 1974, a public hearing with a large audience of community supporters in attendance was held with the Connecticut Commission on Hospitals and Health Care. Many persons stood up to question the need for a hospice facility, asking why existing nursing homes and hospitals couldn't do the job. One influential opponent took the platform to say that a hospice would be unnecessary if the clergy would simply do their jobs well. He accused the clergy of supporting the hospice concept so they could run away from their responsibilities to dying persons. The chairman of the hospice board replied that quite the opposite was true, that the hospice program would provide a way for the clergy to be actively and more deeply involved in teamwork with medical personnel. After physicians, attorneys and other hospice advocates had patiently answered each objection that was raised, licensure was granted as of June 1974, with the understanding that all physicians would have admitting privileges and that patients would be taken regardless of their ability to pay. Asked to share with persons considering hospice programs elsewhere what he learned from these negotiations, the chairman of the board said: "One has to pull together a lot of data to convince such licensing bodies, which are skeptical at first. We were irritated that there seemed to be so many blocks put in our way, but these barriers exist and must be transcended. Maybe these are important to make sure that we are spending enough time in planning, and in education for attitude change. We had to learn to be patient and to move slowly as we built up support."

On May 10, 1974, the New Haven Hospice board of directors announced that it had purchased farm land in Branford, Connecticut; namely, a six-acre site for the facility which was to be constructed. The site is only twelve minutes from the center of New Haven by car, is located on a bus stop, with a school and church across the street, all of which will keep patients from feeling isolated. The purchase, which was completed in December of 1975, was the foundation for facilitating fund-raising from foundations and individuals, and as of November 1978, the state of Connecticut had appropriated $1,500,000 towards the total cost of $3,500,000. The federal government through H.E.W. had appropriated $1,000,000, leaving $1,000,000 which was being raised from the private sector.

Planning the Design

"It is a mistake to think of our hospice as a *place*, a special type of hospital for the dying," the chairman of the board stressed. "Our first emphasis is on home care, on keeping as many patients at home as possible." But at the same time in selecting LoYi Chan as architect the hospice board was opting for a design which would stretch the imagination. The fact that Chan had never designed any sort of hospital and would therefore approach the hospice need with an open mind impressed the Building Committee, which didn't want an architect with preconceived ideas. The chairman of the committee was Henry Wald, director of health-facilities planning at Yale, and the committee was influenced also by John Thompson, hospital design consultant and author of *The Hospital: A Social and Architectural History*, who feels that the old idea of one hospital to satisfy all needs is a thing of the past. While there may always be a need for some "health-care factories" for short-term intensive care, he told Joan Kron, there is a need for facilities where humanity won't have to overcome technical apparatus.[6] LoYi Chan's design for the American hospice gives priority to family needs, instead of excluding them as most hospitals do, and gives attention to psychological and social needs of patient and family.

The architect—from the firm of Prentice and Chan, Olhausen—has designed a 44-bed hospice facility which consists of two V-shaped wings, each having service and administrative rooms at the center. As the patient enters the new facility he will first approach "transition spaces" which will prepare him psychologically and which are designed to relieve anxiety even before one enters the building. The visitor, approaching the hospice, will first of all see the staff dining room and a street-level day-center center for the children of employees, so that as Kron suggests: "Even people driving by the hospice will see that it is not a death house." [7] A visitor will enter through what the architect calls "escape valves"—*i.e.*, antechambers where people can deal with their emotions before they go inside. Patients and visitors will enter the building through the same door, and whatever their emotion may be, the building will welcome them as a homelike, warm place. Next the visitor or patient will move toward one of the wings through a living room with a fireplace, which the architect describes as another "valve" where the visitor can make another step in dealing with his emotions on his way to where the patients live.

Instead of formal corridors as in most hospitals, the Chan design provides for front and back halls—one on each side of the patients' rooms. The back hall will be private, for bathrooms, supply rooms, and staff work space. The front hall, which will greet both patient and guest, will be warmly lighted and spacious, with room for social life and space enough for beds to be rolled there, or out into the garden. Each room will have "greenhouse windows" full of flowering plants, and the patients will always have floods of light and an adequate view of nature outside to keep them closely involved with the rhythm of life. Following the plan of British hospices, the patients will for the most part live in four-bed rooms, which will provide fellowship, enabling patients to support one another. It is not good to die alone, even where the low partitions provide a sense of privacy and continuing supervision. For one patient to be alone as another dies is not good, tensions often arise with three persons—so four has been found to be the ideal number. There will be a number of one-bed rooms, however, for the occasional patient who needs to be alone with wife, family, or with personal problems.

The furnishings will be homey and patients can bring their own possessions from home as they wish. There will be lots of clocks and telephones—so that patients can keep in close touch with their friends. Kitchenettes for private use will enable families to prepare favorite foods, and comforters and spreads on the beds will be handmade. Coffee on the stove will be one of many expressions of the theme: This is a home. One point of discussion led to disagreement with funeral directors who wanted immediately after death to remove the body through a private exit, whereas the hospice directors felt that the body should be kept for a time at the facility so that the family and others could confront death right away to help them adjust to it in a realistic and healthy way. Many studies of the bereavement process, have found that survivors must not be allowed to pretend that the loved one has not died.[8] YoLi Chan therefore designed a unique homey sort of viewing room, where the body will be kept on a bed, rather than in a casket, and where family members or other visitors may sit close or at a distance, in accordance with their emotions.

Hospice staffs both in Britain and America agree that a facility with the wrong sort of staff can accomplish little, no matter how excellent its architecture; and that the right staff people can minister with great effectiveness to the terminally ill amid totally inadequate facilities. The New Haven Hospice sought to construct a model facility, not to overemphasize the importance of a separate building, but because it is felt that an excellent building can make a highly visible contribution to patients who can thrive in pleasant surroundings, as well as serving as a demonstration place and training center for persons who will serve as staff on hospice teams elsewhere. If there is to be a building, therefore, the hospice board feels it must be one in which brick and stone demonstrate and underline the hospice philosophy at every possible point. The facility will symbolize, to the many visitors who come to see it, a vision of new possibilities and important changes which are needed and possible in the American health-care system.

Hospice Home Care

The planners for the New Haven Hospice first assumed that their task was to duplicate in America the sort of hospice facility which had proven so effective in England, but it soon became apparent as they studied the need that the focus in America should first of all be on home care for the terminally ill, with the hospice as backup to the program rather than its center. Home care has been increasingly emphasized in England, but with an excellent facility to work from, it has perhaps not been as apparent to British hospice staffs that most of what needs to be done can quite well be accomplished without the facility. Most patients wish to stay at home as long as they can, to die at home if possible. And even if this were not so, cancer care statistics for 1973 indicate that for patients suffering advanced cancer, average hospital costs were $21,718 per patient; and 30 per cent of them incurred expenses of $25,000 to $50,000 in a period when inflation was continuing to cause regular increases in the spiral of costs.[9] Keeping the dying person at home is not only financially advantageous to the family, the Federal government and the insurance companies but also it enables the terminally ill to escape institutional encroachments upon their dignity, to avoid the isolation and autonomy which is so often their lot, and makes it possible for them to continue sharing in the life of their family.

For example, a retired Navy warrant officer learned that he had terminal cancer. When the family physician suggested a nursing home the patient and his family detested the idea, yet "the children were going to pieces" over his condition. Instead of surrendering to institutional care, however, this patient was able to become related to the New Haven Hospice. Soon he was able to share fully again in the lives of his wife and two sons, free from the pain. "They got me back up; I'm enjoying life again," he told a reporter.[10] Such an incident is possible because the hospice team is providing around-the-clock, seven-days-a-week professional services to aid the family in caring for terminally-ill people at home, which has been too expensive for the majority of families in the past. Thus nearly all of the first seventy-five families in the program of the New Haven Hospice were able to keep their dying family member at home for two to three weeks longer than would otherwise have been possible. Visitors to the New Haven Hospice program now find a situation in which 74 per cent of the hospice patients died at home, surrounded by their families during the twelve months ending September 30, 1978. Sometimes, for example, living on a rented hospital bed in the middle of the living room for as long as three months. By being available on call at all times, the hospice team can relieve not only the pain of the patient but also the exhaustion of the family seeking to take care of a patient. The recovery of mutual health care then possible helps create a happy environment for all. Essential to this home-care program is bereavement care for survivors for a year after death. The hospice staff has discovered a type of care that helps increase the capacity of the patient and his or her family to live through the experience of dying with meaning and dignity, with the total well-being and life-style of each patient seen as central.

Pain Care in America

Not all terminal illness, not even all cancer, produces intense physical pain, but a picture of how pain control can function in the life of a dying person is recorded in detail in Stewart Alsop's book on the last few months of his life.[11] At first the principal difference between British and American pain care with terminally-ill persons seems to be the use of heroin in British medication. And it is true that with the use of heroin against the law in the United States, American medicine has tended not to place as much emphasis on the use of narcotics in pain control, frequently making use of radiotherapy for bony metastases, of anesthetic nerve blocks for neurosurgery, and of physiotherapy. There is an underlying issue of even greater significance, however. As early as 1961, Walter Modell, the director of Clinical Pharmacology at Cornell University, warned that the concentration of American medicine on cure was resulting in a neglect of relieving distress, which he said was hardly being taught to American medical students at all. "My stand," he said, "is that what the symptom causes can be as important as what causes the symptom." [12] The relief of distressing symptoms, therefore, is an urgently important part of medicine and to deprive a patient of pain control is to deprive him of a significant part of what medicine has to offer. Many symptoms, he said, are no longer merely guideposts to follow in search for more serious ailments, but may themselves harm the patient—such, for example, as nausea and pain. The physician has the important responsibility of making the patient more comfortable, which often is an essential precondition to treatment, or is a substitute for it when no treatment is possible.

The Branford Hospice experience in pain control is technically explained to physicians in an article by Dr. Arthur Lipman.[13] Mount and others who have used British pain-control methods in a hospice program in Canada suggest the following aims of treatment for intractable pain in persons who have advanced malignant disease: 1) identify the cause, 2) prevent the pain before it recurs, 3) reduce anxious anticipation and memory of the pain so that the amount of narcotic can be gradually reduced, 4) remove the patient from the perpetual somnolence which so often is the result of sedation for pain, 5) make it possible for the patient to relate to his environment normally, and 6) administer the medication in a way which makes it possible for the patient to retain a degree of independence and mobility, which is not possible when analgesics are given parenterally.[14]

Unfortunately many physicians do not proceed farther than to investigate the effects of the drug, ignoring the effect of the physician's own behavior or factors other than the medication which may be having an effect. Also the physician often overlooks the peculiarities of a specific patient.[15]

Psychological pain also may take many forms and be of any degree of quality, and require psychotherapeutic rather than pharmaceutical treatment. But Modell insisted that it is most important to prevent pain through drug use once it has developed. It is easier to slow down the development of the pain mechanism—"to interrupt or derail the entire train of events involved in pain" [16]—than to suppress or transform the elements once they become fully developed. This is true in part, he says, because once pain has developed to the point of intensity at which there are serious psychological reactions, the relief of a well-developed and powerful experience of pain becomes much more complicated and difficult. Also, once a feeling of pain is communicated by the patient to someone else, Gouda says,[17] it becomes something interpersonal, to be treated on that level, as part of the interrelationship between persons. Psychic factors are seen as often determining the tolerability of pain, for an experience which causes pain in one culture may not be considered painful in another, and pain under terminal conditions is strongly influenced by people's own feelings about death and how it is understood by people around them. Pain may be physically caused, but it may be greatly increased by the encouragement of other individuals who are communicating their fears and anxieties to the dying person.

The New Haven Hospice staff tries to shift the focus of the dying person away from preoccupation with his or her pain, by altering the milieu and the attitudes of the family in order to shift to a positive view of the patient's personal sources of pleasure. The staff team must establish a relationship of trust and win the confidence of the family and friends, so that they feel free to express their fears, feelings, thoughts, and concerns. To accomplish this the staff must be honest, considerate, supportive, and dependable. Whereas many institutions find it essential to ritualize care, thereby often turning it into an impersonal routine; instead of such institutionalization, the hospice team seeks to personalize care and to individualize it.

Although heroin is not available for their use, American hospice programs find quite adequate substitutes when they wish to use a liquid mixture.[16] Sometimes a hospice will have difficulty with drug regulations or enforcers—as, for example, in getting adequate amounts of a drug such as methadone for a patient to use at home. Many American physicians and others concerned have not given adequate attention to research and evaluation of pain-care possibilities such as have been carried out at Royal Victoria Hospital in Montreal.[17] One interesting aspect of this research was the discovery that similar patients given the same medication had less pain in the hospice program than if they were in the wards of the general hospital. This suggests that whether or not the hospices have anything new to teach, the development of the New Haven Hospice as a model can be helpful as a means of calling attention to factors in pain control which have been, and are being, neglected. One of the most effective demonstrations that the New Haven Hospice makes to visiting physicians and others is to let them meet and talk to people whose pain is being controlled. One woman, for example, was in great misery because she wanted to live to see a grandchild about to be born, but knew it was impossible. The controlling of her pain, however, made it possible for her to recover enough strength to knit a gift for the child she would never see, thus helping to brighten her last days. Another hospice patient had been lying all the time in a fetal position with a hot water bottle clutched to his chest, staring into space, moaning in his private hell which he said was compounded by pain which was like fire—as if someone "put a hot iron in your hand." But when the hospice team showed him they could control his pain he became a different person, able to live rather than vegetate during his last days.

What happens without the hospice? In one reported case, for example, a man was brought into a hospital emergency room in excruciating pain. He was very short of breath. The family begged that he be readmitted to the hospital since they could not deal with his pain at home: "We literally begged the physician to admit my brother, but they threw him out. The doctor in Emergency said that there was 'no way'—that we could sue him or the hospital . . . but he was going home. . . . We went home in tears. The next week was hell and finally we had to bring him back. Fortunately there was a new doctor in Emergency and he had my brother admitted. He died four hours later. You know, they simply phoned us that he had died. No word of anything that had been done for him, what he'd said, whether he had been comfortable . . ."[18]

Note: In 1979, Connecticut Hospice, Inc., was adopted as the official name for the Branford Hospice at New Haven.

FOR FURTHER READING

To Honor All of Life, A National Demonstration Center to Protect the Rights of the Terminally Ill, Prospectus of Hospice, Inc., 765 Prospect St., New Haven, Conn., 06511, March 1976; Gibson, Ronald, "Home Care of Terminal Malignant Diseases," *Journal of the Royal College of Surgeons*, January 1971; and on pain-care research: Marks, R. N. and Sacher, F. J., "Undertreatment of Medical Patients with Narcotic Analgesics," *Annals of Internal Medicine*, 78, 193, 1975; Melzack, R. *The Puzzle of Pain.* London: Penguin, 1973; "The McGill Pain Questionnaire," *Pain*, 1975, 1: p. 277; Melzack, R. Ofiesch, J. G., and Mount, B. M., "The Brompton Mixture: Effects on Pain in Cancer Patients," *Canadian Medical Association Journal*, July 17, 1976, p.125; detailed case studies in the *October 1976 Report of the Palliative Care Service of Royal Victoria Hospital, op. cit.*

6

Challenges and Alternatives

No one way to care for dying persons is best for every individual or community. The hospice as specialized institution or program—valuable as it is for experimentation, research, staff training, and as a demonstration model to stimulate like action elsewhere—is challenged by alternative care programs for dying persons. Perhaps the primary North American challenge to the New Haven Hospice as model for other communities is the demonstration of what is possible in a hospice wing or ward of a general hospital, as illustrated by St. Luke's in New York and the Royal Victoria in Montreal. Dr. Balfour Mount, director of the Palliative Care Unit at Royal Victoria, does not "wholly follow St. Christopher's," since he has "serious reservations" as to the extent society can afford to support a sufficient number of separate hospice facilities.[1]

Caring environments for terminally-ill persons could be provided in a variety of settings:

1. The patient might be placed in a unique palliative-care facility like St. Christopher's in London.

2. Similar care and concern might be provided in a special wing or ward of a hospital, such as the Palliative Care Unit at Royal Victoria Hospital.

3. A hospice team might work with terminally-ill persons

on various floors of the hospital, such as at St. Luke's in New York City.

4. A dying patient might be in a place which specializes exclusively in the care of terminally-ill persons, such as Calvary Hospital in the Bronx, New York.

5. Or the patient might be cared for in a nursing home, such as those specialized homes operated by the Sisters of St. Rose Hawthorne in the New York area.

6. The patient might remain at home with special assistance in care provided for the family by a team of home-visiting specialists.

7. A day-care institution for the terminally ill might be developed to provide a combination of home care and an inpatient facility where needed.

8. There are radical experiments at creating a unique environment for dying persons through the use of LSD, hypnotism, "inner environment" religious experiences through Yoga and meditation—one or another of these may be combined with psychiatry.

9. Other new alternatives may well emerge.

Criteria for Evaluation

Yeates Conwell, in pointing out the deficiency of present care in most communities and the lack of adequate alternatives,[2] proposes ten criteria for use in deciding which alternatives provide the best care for the terminally ill:

1. For good terminal care the delivery system must have a set of standards upon which to structure and evaluate its caring function. There is evidence that the lack of agreed-upon standards contributes to the unacceptable level of care which is frequently observed.

2. Care must be patient centered; respecting, for example, a patient's ethnic differences and tradition, including his ideas about illness, death and dying.

3. The patient should have the opportunity to discuss death and dying, with people available who are capable and willing to take up the challenge to help the patient work through this difficult period.

4. There should be a team approach to terminal care, and the team/patient relationship should be mutually supportive and continuous.

5. The care system must facilitate the interaction of patient, family, and friends, including support for the family until death occurs and providing bereavement care afterward.

6. Patients should be provided with the opportunity to keep their own clothes and other personal possessions, as a symbol of continuity with their previous life-style and to maintain strands of normalcy in life.

7. Persons should be helped to die where they wish, whether in a facility or at home, and the caring system should co-operate in providing access to programs and facilities best suited to their individual needs.

8. Pain must be effectively and sensitively controlled.

9. The treatment philosophy must respect the rights of the patient as earlier described.

10. Good terminal care should be financially available to everyone.

There was a danger that the term *hospice* might be used for any sort of ill-run commercial establishment which wanted to profit from care of the terminally ill, so a move is under way in 1976–77 to establish standards and an agreed-upon definition of a hospice.[3] Representatives of various hospice programs are beginning to meet to define their nature and obligations. Pending completion of the task of establishing criteria, the term *hospice* is subject to abuse by correspondence school certification and low-quality programs. Its best sources of criteria were the experience of individual hospice programs, such as those defined by the New Haven Hospice. With respect to the needs of the patient, the following criteria were provisionally proposed:

—availability and accessibility of care,

—effectiveness of pain and symptom relief management,

—freedom from unnecessary dependency and assistance in adjusting to necessary dependency,

—sense of continuing self-respect and identity as a person,

—sense of control and involvement in decision-making,

—continuing meaningful social activity,

—freedom from fear of abandonment or social isolation,

—freedom from financial insecurity and from being a burden—financial or physical, or emotional—on the family,

—sense of continued belief in the meaningfulness and quality of life,

—maintenance of honest relationships without fear and without expressing either positive or negative emotions.

The following additional criteria were proposed with respect to the needs of the patient's family:

—availability and accessibility of care,

—help with the physical burdens of care,

—continuing of relationship and openness of communication with the care-giving team,

—sense of participation in care-giving and decision-making,

—free access to the patient,

—availability of assistance in adjusting to impending death (an outlet for grief, help with fear of loss, resentments, guilt, etc.) during bereavement period.

General Hospital: A Sobering Project in Self-Analysis

At present most terminally-ill people are scattered around in various wards of hospitals. Perhaps the most careful research on their care was that undertaken at Royal Victoria Hospital in Montreal as part of an assessment which led to the establishment of a Palliative Care Unit in that 1,000-bed referral and teaching hospital at McGill University. In the early 1970's, serious questions were raised about the treatment of terminally-ill persons in the hospital; and in 1972 a research program gathered data upon which changes might be proposed, concentrating on case studies and questionnaires. A 21-question instrument was given to all members of the health-care staff—orderlies, for example, as well as nurses and physicians. Patients were also questioned to discover discrepancies between physician and patient in their perception of attitudes and treatment. The survey found wide differences between what the patients actually thought, and what physicians had perceived them as thinking. For example, did patients want to know the truth about their prognosis? Only 43 per cent of the physicians thought that terminally-ill patients wanted to know; whereas 64 per cent of the patients said they did want to know. One of the significant aspects of the study was the fact that of 700 nurses, only 225 were interested enough to fill out the questionnaire; and of 340 resident and intern physicians, only 91. For the most part the staff was found to be complacent and satisfied with things as they were. Yet when the questionnaire returns and case studies were analyzed, more than 200 deficiencies in the hospital's system for caring for the terminally ill were defined.[4] For example, it was found that staff relationships with patients were too impersonal, that the family of the patient was frequently excluded from discussion, that doctors and nurses avoided the terminally ill, that the medical staff was uncomfortable and embarrassed when a patient wanted to discuss his or her forthcoming death. Further, there was over-investigation and overtreatment of the critically ill; the staff lacked expertise in dealing with emotional needs of dying persons; there were multiple communication gaps between doctor-nurse-patient-family-clergy-social worker, and so on; relatives were excluded at time of death; there were bilingual communication gaps; there were no private or peaceful places on the ward for in-depth talks with patient and family, and terminally-ill patients were often isolated. The hospital staff appeared to see few of these problems.

The most persuasive part of the research, however, were the

case studies of specific patients—stories painstakingly gathered by medical students who were free to linger around the wards to watch and to talk with the patients. Detailed notes were taken on specific cases, such as 80-year-old Miss R who was in the hospital for thirty-five days as a terminal patient.[5] She was isolated behind drawn curtains, and when the interviewer intruded, she pleaded: "Please come talk to me." During her 35-day stay in the hospital she was cared for by 38 different nurses. Except for three days in July Miss R was never cared for by the same nurse on two consecutive days. Of the 105 nursing shifts during her hospital stay, the nurses recorded her status only for 66 shifts, and only nine of the nurses' notes mentioned her psychological pain, that she was very lonely, crying all day, depressed, asking to die, afraid of everything. Because she was continually calling for a nurse to rectify her isolation, nurses responded to her call bell with increasing delay, avoiding her as much as possible. The resident physicians on ward rounds were found to spend only an average of one minute in Miss R's room, none got close enough to touch her, and only rarely did anyone speak to her. She begged the student observer to stay with her, after he held her hand and listened to her talk. She pleaded: "Help me, you are not like the others, help me." The staff laughed nervously in discussing the fact that she once called the police for help. She voiced suicidal thoughts of trying to jump out the window, and the staff reaction was an expressed wish to get her moved out of the ward to a nursing home, because they found her care so troublesome.

The result of such stories was an explosive report, which caused one physician to say: "The editor of the *Journal of the American Medical Association* who said in 1974 that there was no problem had obviously not seen this report or read these stories." Why had problems of such dimensions crept into the hospital care of the terminally ill? One interpreter of the Royal Victoria data said that health-care professionals are suffering from future shock as a result of the explosion in medical information and knowledge. The inevitable result is more and more specialization, with fewer and fewer physicians having time for personal relationships with a patient. "Of course, we physicians understand ourselves to be compassionate," he said. "So we never see where we are falling down and the hospital is failing the terminally ill—the cracks in the system." The specialist always wants to keep "doing his thing," never ceasing his efforts to prolong life in case something has been missed. "These, and ill-informed attitudes toward pain control, are reasons why general hospitals are bad places, increasingly, for terminally-ill people."

The Specialized Hospital

Calvary Hospital, operated by the Roman Catholic Archdiocese in New York City, is for patients who are medically indigent, have cancer, and have a life expectancy of three to six weeks. Most of its patients are referred to Calvary from other acute-care hospitals, and the proof that most are unable to pay is demonstrated by the fact that nearly 60 per cent of Calvary's operating income is from Medicaid and most of the remaining 40 per cent from Medicare. The aim of the 75-year-old 110-bed facility is "to give patients the best quality of life possible during their last days and help them die with dignity and grace; clean, out of pain, and if possible with all fear of death removed." [6] To achieve this the Calvary staff has developed a philosophy it calls "an integrated approach to death," in which the medical and nursing staffs, the Protestant and Catholic chaplains and visiting clergy, and the social-service staff work together to meet the physical, spiritual, and psychological needs of the dying. On the average two people die at Calvary Hospital each day, or $\frac{1}{35}$th of all cancer deaths in the New York area each year.[7] The medical staff consists of five full-time internists, each with a subspecialty; nursing is provided by the Sisters of the Little Company of Mary, a Catholic order which is involved in forty-two hospitals and mission clinics in various countries; and nurse's aides—called "cancer care technicians" because of their skill and training—who are reputedly very proficient. In co-operation with three medical schools, Calvary Hospital conducts training programs with a summer "extern" program for a hundred or so students, partly to change the attitudes of future physicians toward the terminally ill.

Beginnings have been made in bereavement care for families who solicit such assistance, and the hospital insists upon a close physician-patient relationship as well as a strong bond between patients and other members of the staff. One Calvary patient, found crying, was asked what was wrong. "What's wrong," she replied. "I've been in hospitals for two years and that's the first time anyone ever called me by name." Each patient is assigned to a specific physician, and channels of open communication guarantee that patient and family can establish a positive and personal relationship. One fundamental difference between Calvary and the British hospice model is that while no one can be admitted to Calvary Hospital until he or she has been dismissed by previous physicians, Calvary does undertake more than palliative care. Every new patient, upon admission at Calvary, is put through a new clinical evaluation to make sure that no curative possibilities have been overlooked. Calvary Hospital is primarily interested in the medical management of advanced cancer patients, but at times a weakness in the patient's previous treatment is uncovered and it is then corrected by active therapeutic measures. "A dying patient often takes a renewed interest in life," one of the administrators of the hospital said, "when he finds people genuinely concerned about him." But, while chemotherapy, and so on, may be initiated at times, no use is made of "heroic measures" —cardiac defibrillators and such—so in this way Calvary's philosophy is similar to the hospice concept.

Should terminally-ill persons everywhere be sent to such

specialized hospitals? In most areas, such specialized institutions would remove patients too far from their families. Also, Calvary Hospital does not find it possible to offer the range of services which are provided by St. Christopher's or the New Haven Hospice in, for example, home-care services or bereavement counseling. And some critics are convinced that the specialty hospital will in most places continue to be a large, impersonal place, despite some excellent exceptions like Calvary, for not all can be operated by church orders and with such a hospice-type philosophy without radical changes in standards and procedures.

A Special Nursing Home

"Where," we asked a hospital administrator, "can a terminally-ill patient be sent with the confidence that he or she will get excellent care—if, for example, the patient has no family?" The administrator replied: "We wish there were more nursing homes like St. Rose's." Like Calvary Hospital, the homes operated by the Sisters of St. Rose Hawthorne, founded under impetus from the daughter of Nathaniel Hawthorne, are church-related institutions which have sought to care for poor persons who have incurable cancer. While not meeting many of the criteria proposed by Conwell, these homes do suggest that in many smaller communities a nursing home might be especially equipped to perform some hospice functions in cooperation with a team of professionals and volunteers in the community. As in the hospice concept, the Catholic sisters who operate these five nursing homes, largely in the New York City area, have created a unique caring environment wherein patients are encouraged to help take care of one another and support one another. The most striking feature to observers is the cheerfulness of patients and staff alike, who bring a spirit of joy into the midst of death with the philosophy that "a sympathetic nurse with tender hands can do more to relieve all that discourages peace of mind . . . than can any opiate." [8]

Radical Environments

At the opposite extreme from traditional religious institutions are some current experiments at creating new environments for the terminally ill through the use of sound and light—some even dream of laser projectors that will transform a dying patient's wall into a splashing waterfall or the roaring waves of the ocean, or an art gallery, concert or a sports event, with an electronic control panel to enable the patient to compose or synthesize a variety of sounds and images into any sort of environment or experience desired. Jerome Singer suggests, indeed, that "fantasies and daydreams, far from being irrelevant and insubstantial, may be the foundation of serenity and purpose in our lives." [9] At the Maryland Psychiatric Center near Baltimore, LSD and other psychedelic drugs have been used in experiments to provide supportive therapy for dying persons. Patients have been helped to have beautiful experiences of transcendence and exaltation to "widen the 'broad spectrum of consciousness' which has steadily been narrowing in a scientific age." [10] The inner environment of dying persons has been expanded, and enriched with experiences of exotic color and emotion which have transfigured their time of dying. The patients tell their life story and are helped to sense a creative mystical apprehension of life full of rich meaning, liberating and inspiring the consciousness to soaring flight as reflection and remembrance come together to heal and bring wholeness to the dying experience.

While the present generation of terminally-ill persons probably does not include many who wish such psychedelic experiences, futurists suggest that someday each dying person can have a tailor-made experience, perhaps spending his or her last weeks with family films and tapes which review the person's life, drawing together reflective, mystical and fantasy experience as wished—the "caring team" will include not only physicians, nurses and the present hospice members but also media specialists, music specialists,[11] experts in Yoga, Zen or meditation, and so on. And whatever climactic experiences a dying person might want could well be provided in his or her own home.

One-Person Team

More in keeping with the hospice concept is the work of one nurse in a Pennsylvania hospital who gradually became concerned with her own treatment of terminally-ill persons. For example, she would promise to return to a person who was dying as soon as she finished certain essential jobs with other patients, and then she would find that the patient had died before she was able to return. It distressed the nurse that patients died alone, so she requested permission from the hospital administration to devote her ministrations to a case load of only twelve patients a week, in order that more time and continuity could be given to the terminally ill. Her work has demonstrated that hospice principles can be helpful even when applied by only one nurse within a general hospital's intensive care unit. When she was granted permission to give special attention to the dying, she found that her most important nursing responsibility changed. She became an advocate and a listener, to find out what the dying person wanted. A blind five-year-old boy, for example, wanted to feel a kitten. Nurses are not ordinarily involved in gross rule-breaking, but even though it was against the rules to bring animals into the hospital, that child had his kitten before he died. The nurse "bent" the rules to adjust them to the needs of the terminally ill. For example, an old man wanted to wear his trousers instead of a hospital gown, so she let him wear his trousers.

"I'm angry," she said, "that so many of our problems with the terminally ill are purely ethical. A physician isn't necessarily more of an expert on ethical issues than anyone else. I'm angry over costs: $50 for a nurse to visit a home just to wash a patient's back and give her some soup. I do get emotionally involved with dying patients. I hug some of them, although with others it isn't appropriate. I give them my home phone number, privately, so that members of the family can telephone me if I am needed during my off hours. It matters how people die. We don't have the right to make decisions for other people about what is important to them. One needs to honor small requests." For example, this "death-and-dying nurse" had a patient who wanted to leave the hospital and die at home. So the nurse taught the patient's husband to administer morphine, a hospital bed was procured, an ambulance was called, and the nurse swiped a few daffodils to send home with the patient. A few days later, on a home visit, the patient was found sleeping, not in the hospital bed, but with her husband. She was retaining food in ways she had not been able to do at the hospital. She no longer needed the morphine, and her husband had been able to take her out into the garden, as she wished, for a last visit there before she died.

Hospice Team in a General Hospital

If one nurse with the hospice concept can make a big difference in a hospital, then much more can be accomplished by a coordinated team of persons working to implement the hospice point of view: physician, nurse, chaplain, social worker, volunteers and others. St. Luke's Hospital in New York City has developed a "hospice team" which specializes in palliative care. The team takes over much of the care for a limited group of terminally-ill persons on a number of different floors in the hospital. At first, members of the team experimented with working in the entire hospital, but in 1976 found that they were working beyond their capacity, for the team was not large enough to deal with the entire hospital complex. By working with patients on certain floors only—in contrast to establishing a "dying ward"—the hospice team has demonstrated methods of care to the entire hospital staff, showing how it is possible to provide a "hospice-type environment" within a large metropolitan hospital.

There is a plan at St. Luke's to remodel a wing of the existing hospital into a hospice unit, so that at least some patients can have the advantages of each other's company and support as in a British hospice. A modest remodeling plan, prepared by a young architect who consulted with the designer of the New Haven Hospice, would incorporate many of the attractive features of a special facility. Construction and land costs are so high in New York City that it would be difficult to secure funds sufficient to construct hospice facilities with gardens and other special features of St. Christopher's Hospice. But a floor of a hospital could be arranged with a kitchenette, space for families, an area for recreation, outpatients, and so on. The hospice concept at St. Luke's, however, takes shape as a special team of persons. There are three nurses (clinical specialists), only one of whom actually gave full time to the hospice program in the fall of 1976. She functioned as an enabler to mobilize the skills of any needed persons from the hospital staff. By maintaining liaison with all departments any needed resource could immediately be brought to bear upon the needs of a dying patient. At the same time the hospice staff made progress in changing the attitudes of the entire hospital staff, and the environment itself, by demonstrating what could be done with the limited resources available.

The hospice team does not immediately take over a case once the physician has assessed the illness to be terminal. First of all the team seeks to establish an advocate-support relationship with the patient and with all the staff on the patient's floor: the nurses, clerk on the floor, aides, housekeeping staff, and any others who will deal with the dying person. The hospice team helps interpret the needs of the terminally-ill patient to these staff people, and supports them in efforts to develop the needed point of view toward death, as well as

proper attitudes toward the patient's family. Instead of conflict developing between the hospice team and the floor staff,
it thus becomes a learning experience for all, rather than "a
case of the hospice team seeming to step in to tell them how to
do their jobs." Most members of a hospital staff feel overworked and in need of more help. Therefore, if the hospice
team lays the right groundwork, and good relationships are
established with the floor staff, there need not be resentment
when the team members offer to provide help and supportive
services. Instead of being critical of other staff members if
they find a dying patient being neglected, the hospice team
expands the scope of its own personal care to the patient as
a help to the overworked staff.

The St. Luke's hospice team has the policy, for example, of
continuing to talk to a patient even after the dying person
appears to be unconscious, for they know that such patients
often can hear what is being said and are reassured by the
presence of a familiar voice. Such talk is more meaningful, of
course, if the team has earlier established a continuing relationship of such conversation with the patient. A greater
degree of continuity thus becomes possible than would otherwise be the case. The hospice team at St. Luke's has also
succeeded in getting many hospital rules relaxed so that terminally-ill patients can have the same privileges they would
enjoy in a separate hospice facility: unlimited visitors, the
presence of children and pets, overnight room and board pro-
visions for family members, a shampoo without doctor's
orders, time in the cathedral garden, even a birthday party for
twenty guests. The team not only serves as advocate for the
patient to the hospital administration but also as advocates
for the hospice concept, finding that physicians are more
easily persuaded by demonstration than by arguments. Instead
of taking over care of the patient, the team seeks to work with
all nurses and patients so that they can be involved in new
ways of working and caring. The aim is not to create a team

of specialists in care for the dying, but to correct deficiences in the health-care system.

A major difference between the New Haven Hospice and the St. Luke's hospice team is that of 175 terminally-ill patients who have been involved with the St. Luke's team, as of November 1976, only four died at home. In part, while St. Luke's home-care staff seek to facilitate a home-care effort, these statistics are felt to reflect in part the nature of Manhattan Island. It is one thing for a middle-class suburban patient who has a lovely house and garden to want to die at home, but St. Luke's Hospital is surrounded by a community of poverty where many elderly patients live in a dingy room up six flights of stairs—or so many family members may be crowded in a few rooms that it is simply not feasible for a patient to have palliative care at home.

Palliative Care Unit in a Large Hospital

The case studies and questionnaire research which revealed serious discrepancies in the care of terminally-ill persons at Royal Victoria Hospital in Montreal were persuasive with the officials whose authorization was needed for experimentation with a pilot project to establish a Palliative Care Unit. A ward was set aside for terminally-ill patients and a team was assigned to work there, completing a chain of events which began with a seminar on death and dying held in February of 1973. For the initial two-year period the experiment was limited to patients whose physicians certified that they could not be cured. The basic aim of the unit was palliative—to lengthen the time of survival and to enhance its quality. It was soon discovered by the hospice team at Royal Victoria Hospital that curable patients could cause as much difficulty in the ward for dying persons as the terminally-ill people did in other wards. Some people were, of course, reluctant at first to be moved into a "dying ward" until they saw what a pleasant place it was with its emphasis upon good nursing and pain control. Most important, perhaps, was the word that "there is no parking meter on the bed"—*i.e.*, patients could remain as long as they needed care without needing to worry that the hospital would dismiss them because cure was no longer possible. There were continuing problems, of course. The director said: "How do you explain to hospital colleagues that the presence of a pet dog or cat may be more relevant than arterial blood gases?" The usual hospital rules were altered, as in a British hospice, to allow children and families a continuing role in the lives of patients. Special volunteers were sought—including, for example, a woman professor of philosophy with great spiritual depth. There were volunteers who were ready to listen to patients and to understand them as they were, rather than as someone thought they ought to be. Morning and evening prayers were introduced into a secular institution, which even atheist and agnostic patients found to be important—for their neighbors if not for themselves, in a context where patients took an interest in helping one another. "Teamwork," the director said, "doesn't just happen. It requires continuing effort." In the October 1976 report of the Palliative Care Unit, he said: "Those who have been involved have grown immeasurably. We have learned a great deal from our patients. We have been heartened by the capacity for growth in time of adversity and by man's willingness to give to his fellow man when the opportunity is provided. It has been a rare privilege to take part in the first tottering steps of an infant discipline." [12]

At the end of the two-year pilot project, a careful evaluation was undertaken. An impressive group of international consultants were invited to Montreal and were given copies of the 516-page research document.[13] The conclusion was "that the care of the dying and their families can be greatly improved. The cost involved is minimal—insignificant in the light of the suffering alleviated. There is, in fact, a saving in costs per patient treated," as a Palliative Care Unit makes it possible for more patients to die at home and frees active treatment beds in an acute hospital. The hard-won expertise of the general hospital—to investigate, diagnose, cure—and the needs of terminally-ill persons are mismatched, the study decided, resulting in compounded suffering. With "caring attention to detail," the Palliative Care Unit had achieved important advances in the standards of medical care. "The use of intravenous fluids and nasogastric tubes has largely been abandoned and with few exceptions intractable pain is controlled without sedation or other undesirable effects, such as personality change." Speaking of a typical case, the report notes: "When Mrs. T died on the Unit, the staff realized that their presence had transformed her agony into peace. She in turn took comfort in the knowledge that she had given as much as she had received." [14]

One of the principal aims of the Palliative Care Unit is to encourage study and education to further understanding of concepts in terminal care, with "conferences, lectures, seminars, discussion groups, workshops, service rounds, student electives and option courses, residency rotations, in-service education." [15] And the consultation team of the Unit acts as a resource within the whole hospital, working in concert with physicians and nurses to counsel them on the care of terminal patients wherever they may be, with specific suggestions for the management of troublesome symptoms or to help them with family or psychological problems. In conclusion, the report not only urged the continuation and growth of the palliative care service at Royal Victoria Hospital but also recommended that similar services be developed throughout Canada as soon as possible. More specifically it was recommended that the Palliative Care Unit be accorded status within the Department of Surgery and that the patients admitted to its care be "those for whom cure and prolongation of life are no longer valid treatment goals, but for whom therapy aimed at improving the quality of the remaining life is appropriate for both patients and their families." [16] It was further recommended that the Palliative Care Unit be expanded to a 30- or 40-bed facility, so that up to 20 per cent of patients there could be "long-stay" patients. Admission to the Unit would be determined by the Palliative Care physician and Admission Committee, with first priority being given to oncology patients already in the hospital. It was recommended that the home-care program of the Unit be continued in association with the Department of Community Health in the city, with home-care nurses trained in the skills of physical diagnosis and symptom control. The recommendations included a proposal that a bereavement follow-up group be established which would include a social worker, psychiatrist, chaplain, nurses, and trained volunteers. More attractive physical surroundings were recommended, with careful attention to be paid to lighting, colors, hand rails, and so on.

It is evident that Royal Victoria's Palliative Care Unit proposes a comprehensive model for work with terminally-ill patients in a hospital. The Unit had not, as of September 1976, received any of the promised funding from the province of Quebec and was being financed through the hospital budget, with research, administration, teaching, and developmental costs in the budget being funded by foundations and special individual gifts. The social worker's salary was paid by the Ville Marie Social Service Center. There had been no special hospice chaplain at Royal Victoria, and the Catholic, Anglican, and United Church chaplains of the hospital had not been able to give as much time to the Unit as they would have wished, because of pressing duties in the entire institution. A visitor to the 12-bed Unit first of all noticed that the physical facilities were far from ideal. The Unit team had to begin with the sort of ward one might find in any hospital, and thereby demonstrate what might be done in any hospital without the expense of remodeling. Quarters were not adequate, but the waiting room was adapted for family and recreational use, and the emphasis on personal care transcended the limitations. If Elisabeth Kübler-Ross is able to recommend the Royal Victoria hospice unit as "an example of the best total care on the continent," it is partly because of the thoroughness in research and quality of care which is everywhere evident, and which is rooted in the conviction that "it's the quality of life that matters."

Separate Facility vs. Hospital Ward

The evidence is not yet conclusive as to whether separate hospices should be advocated or whether communities should be urged to develop hospice teams within existing hospitals. The completion of the New Haven Hospice, which can be studied as a model, will provide some of the needed evidence. Initially, however, in advance of conclusive facts, it is clear that the answer may be different for one community from that for another. Some areas of the country which simply have a population too small to sustain a separate facility can apply the hospice concept through the adaptation of some existing nursing-home and hospital facilities to care for those terminally-ill patients who cannot remain at home until death. In the large urban area of New York City, some patients have preferred to die at St. Luke's, for example, because the hospital has much more pleasant surroundings than their sixth-floor walkup with falling plaster. The impressive arguments which hospice team members at St. Luke's or Royal Victoria Hospital present for working within the structure of existing institutions seems at each point, however, to be refuted by counter-evidence from those who advocate separate hospices. For example:

When patients go to a hospice facility they may lose touch with the family physician and specialists who have been responsible up to that point. It is argued that even when a family physician is highly interested in maintaining the relationship, he does not have the time to do so when the patient is discharged from his care and is no longer in the hospital he regularly visits. On the other hand, such a continuing interest of the physician when the patient is at the hospital is an argument for removing the patient to a hospice if the previous physician disagrees with and interferes in the work of the hospice staff. The instructions of the hospice staff have been interfered with in home care. In a separate institution this sort of conflict is less likely.

It is argued that the hospital provides vastly more resources to be drawn upon by the hospice team than would be available in a separate facility. On the other hand, the terminally-ill patient does not need to pay a share for all the unneeded services and equipment, the very existence of which may at times tempt a resident physician to undertake "heroic measures" or to experiment with the dying patient by trying out new curative treatments.

It is argued that the basic need is for tender loving care, and that the right kind of staff team can provide excellent hospice care wherever the patient is—in hospital as well as in a special hospice facility. However, it is often so difficult to change procedures and attitudes in an existing institution—hospital procedures and practices being so habitual and ingrained—that a new type of facility is needed for the terminally ill. No matter how much a hospital may change in appearance, environment, and staff attitudes, it carries a heavy psychological burden of attitudes in the public mind, whereas a new type of facility can establish an entirely different sort of public image. One has only to contrast LoYi Chan's architectural vision with the best hospitals to understand why one hospice physician tells how, in her anger, she wanted to break the hermetically sealed windows of a hospital room when a dying patient asked for a whiff of the fresh spring air.

Inasmuch as the staff is the key to success in any hospice program, there are implicit dangers, some feel, if the hospice program is subject to a hospital administration which is complex and changing. When there were changes in the hospital board and administration, the director of one special hospital unit, for example, had to engage in frequent political battles to keep his space, even though the unit had a written agreement. Politically speaking, the hospital like all institutions was controlled by persons with their own priorities when space or financing becomes tight. Any hospital must from time to time re-examine its priorities, must shift staff, must work economies, and face the fact that hospital priorities belong to programs that cure. A separate hospice with its own board could give priority to the terminally ill, under such circumstances, since it would have an administration with a different basic commitment. The separate hospice institution would be less complex.

On the other hand, a physician on a hospital-related palliative care team argues that such difficulties are caused for the most part by the newness of the concept. He predicts that within twenty years Palliative Care Units will be as common and accepted in hospitals as are cardiac units today. Nurses do not have to be rotated out of hospice units, he says, but can have permanent assignments just as they do in operating rooms, cardiac units, and other places in the hospital where specialized training is required. A physician responsible for another sort of special unit, which presumably had acceptance and administrative support, said that despite written agreements and recognition of the importance of the unit, he had difficulty keeping key staff when, for example, the director of nursing felt they were temporarily needed elsewhere in the hospital. He said that in a large hospital one cannot change the attitudes and inform all employees and other patients. Perhaps nurses and doctors had a changed attitude toward patients on the special floor, but not all the custodians or people in the finance office, or those who answered telephones had changed their attitudes. There was also subtle pressure from senior staff, who in theory supported the special unit but felt that funds were more needed for new technological equipment when financial shortages forced a battle over priorities. Especially with reference to finances, there were continuing conflicts between physicians who worked in various programs which operated to the detriment of those who were not basically working to cure. So it was increasingly difficult to get the right internes and residents.

Finally the arguments resolve into simple questions: (*a*) How to change the system, and (*b*) How best to serve terminally-ill people. Some of the issues will not be resolved until laws and reimbursement polices are changed. For example, one physician said: "A separate facility might be ideal, but we must at present keep our terminally-ill patients scattered all over the hospital to hide from Federal authorities the fact that we are accepting funds for their care to which we are not technically entitled." Another physician related to a hospice program at a hospital said: "We have to lie a little by not making it clear in our records that Patient X is terminally ill. Otherwise Blue Cross or his insurance company would not pay full rates. They would insist, rather, that the patient be dismissed from the hospital if he or she can no longer be cured."

Perhaps the most convincing arguments for a separate hospice facility are financial: When it is costing up to $80,000 per bed to add hospital space, how can a hospital justify charging less to terminally-ill patients? The answer is that a hospice facility, not having to finance expensive lifesaving equipment, does not have to amortize the cost of that technology by a charge against each bed, and therefore can charge less per day. Even greater savings are possible from taking care of a patient at home. A hospital, for example—such as Royal Victoria—can operate as effective and inexpensive a home-care program for the terminally ill as is possible in relation to a separate facility.

Our conclusion here, nevertheless, is that some separate facilities are now needed, to give leverage and flexibility to the demonstration of hospice methods, and as a base to change the health care system as a whole. Certainly such change must take place from within, and it is therefore perhaps fortunate that excellent hospice programs are currently taking shape both within and outside the hospital. Those who argue that it is nearly impossible to change the attitudes of young physicians (who gain a strong bias in teaching hospitals where they are trained) provide evidence that a separate hospice facility is necessary—at least in current initial stages—so that future hospice staffs can be carefully recruited and trained. Otherwise, they say, an effective demonstration will not be possible or at best will be diluted and overlooked within the large institution. On the other hand, there are those who argue that more change is already taking place than anyone would have expected, as a result of demonstration at places like St. Luke's or Royal Victoria Hospital, and can present impressive evidence that a new climate, with concomitant significant changes in attitude toward death and dying, is rapidly facilitating change.

Long-Range Goals

Long-range goals are approximately the same, among both those who favor hospice units in hospitals and those who favor separate hospice institutions. Nearly all agree that in the long run the entire health-care system will need to adjust itself to provide hospice-type care for terminally-ill persons wherever they are in the system. Visiting nurses, for example, pioneered in basic aspects of hospice-type care. And today in many areas public health and visiting nurses are already changing their procedures to provide hospice-type home care whenever funding programs make it possible for them to expand their staffs. In some areas now the local Visiting Nurse Association has health aides in terminal care, has added social workers, occupational therapists, phychiatrists, and varied resources to its staff and programs so that it can provide hospice-type care for patients and bereavement care for families. As visiting nurses find funding to provide, as hospice teams do, 24-hours-a-day, 7-days-a-week consultation and help with home care, hospice-type services can be extended even into sparsely settled rural areas, so that more and more terminally-ill people can remain at home. Hospice-type programs then will need not be limited to communities large enough to have a general hospital or specialized hospice facility.

At the same time hospitals are also changing, and no one now knows how radically they will continue to change in the next decade under the twin pressures of increasing technology and spiraling costs. Already there are hospitals that have "nursing home" wings—especially some church-related hospitals in the Midwest and West. Hospice teams in those communities may find it easier, as a natural extension of existing health-care facilities, to co-ordinate and transform existing services—as visiting nurse programs, for example, work in liaison with several institutions in the Boston area. Dr. Melvin Krant, who has a high regard for British hospices, has been involved—as director of cancer programs at the new University of Massachusetts School of Medicine in Worcester—in the evaluation of various programs for the terminally ill. In connection with this, he has said: "My first reaction (to the hospice concept) is that it is going to fail as an American idea. It will get into operation, but its intent will fail." [17] Why? He worries that hospices will simply add to the excessive fragmentation, over-specialization and accompanying discontinuity which already plague American medicine. What is needed, he suggests, is integration. He worries also that instead of changing the attitudes of hospitals and physicians, the hospice movement may simply relieve them from the burden of responsibilities they are reluctant to accept: *i.e.*, more community involvement, more basic personal concern for patients.

Certainly the challenge to the medical establishment has come from separate hospice institutions in Britain, but many of the arguments apply to a separate facility, not to a separate institution and program which could preserve its integrity and flexibility to challenge the health-care system. It is argued that this challenge cannot easily be heard within the complex hospital institution, especially the hospice point of view which would give much more freedom to terminally-ill people—not all of whom are old. Indeed, the dying persons with the most difficult problems are those in their thirties and forties with young children and whose youth and health means that it may take them long months or even years to die. Dr. Kübler-Ross proposes that even terminally-ill children should be encouraged to have a positive attitude toward death by being taught how to die. "I even urge them to give away their favorite belongings to those they want to have them," she has said. "I put them in charge of their own deaths." [18]

How can the bureaucratic, technological, mass-treatment hospital understand and accept the implications of such a point of view? Perhaps the best possibility within the near future is to create a variety of institutions for terminally-ill people so that those who wish to do so may have some choice among alternatives. And the separate hospice institution—with or without its separate facility—perhaps with only some leased beds in another type of facility, seems required at this time if any impact is to be made upon the total health-care system . . . and if long-range changes are to be encouraged in the treatment of the terminally ill.

FOR FURTHER READING

Cartwright, A. *et al. Life Before Death.* London: Routledge and Kegan Paul, 1973; Duff, R. S. *et al.*, "Dying and Death," in *Sickness and Society.* New York: Harper and Row, 1968; Gavey, C. J. *The Management of the Hopeless Case.* London: Lewis, 1952; Holford, J. M. "Terminal Care," *Nursing Times,* Jan. 27, 1975; Mount, B. M. "Improving Our Canadian Way of Dying," *Ont. Psychol,* 7: 19, 1975; Smith, S. L., "Care of the Dying," *Lancet,* March 1973; Phillips, D. F., "The Hospital and the Dying Patient," *Hospitals,* February 1972.

7

The Hospice Concept as Program

Whether a hospice is a separate institution or a unit of a hospital, much of what is done is the same—defined at St. Luke's Hospital, for example, as replacing "standard, aggressive medical regimens aimed at cure" which often detract from the quality of life of terminally-ill patients, with a more positive treatment which has two basic aims: 1) "to focus on the real needs of the cancer patient and those close to him in order to enable him to maintain the fullest possible life, and 2) to educate the medical community in alternate methods of caring for these patients." [1] Hospice care is aimed at symptom control, which includes four kinds of pain—physical, psychological, social, and spiritual—nausea and vomiting, weakness, loss of appetite, abdominal distention, and dyspnea. In some cases a patient's life can be extended, and in most cases the quality of a patient's life can be improved. The St. Luke's hospice team has stated the following as its goals:

—to assist patients into a state where they experience relief from distressing symptoms, pain and fear of pain,
—to achieve objective signs in patients indicating feelings of peace and security,
—to review patients weekly in team conferences to determine if goals of hospice care are appropriate,

—to ensure that patients experience increased contact with staff and volunteers as death approaches if they want and need it,

—to give patients and family the opportunity to draw closer together as death approaches,

—to support families in the bereavement process,

—to educate and assist staff in developing an awareness of their own response to death,

—to offer staff the support of the Hospice Team and Hospice Committee as they work with the dying,

—to develop and maintain a program of continuing education and research for hospital staff,

—to provide staff who can support the patient and family through the grief and bereavement process." [2]

How to Accomplish Objectives

A program can easily be described, as in this chapter, but on paper the hospice type of program does not look terribly different from what has been attempted by many agencies in one place or another. The attitude and point of view which underlie and pervade the hospice program are difficult to put on paper or sometimes even for a visitor to see. The Palliative Care Unit at Royal Victoria Hospital dates its beginning to a Task Force on Grief which was formed in February of 1973, and which in turn led to the formation of a Committee on Thanatology—a multidisciplinary committee on death with the assignment of studying the limitations and failures of health care to the terminally ill. In preliminary research and program, significant hospice programs are all *team efforts* and the teams as well as hospice administrative boards are effectively interdisciplinary. The teams attempt to draw together and co-ordinate the planning and work of all persons who have contact with the terminally ill in each specific case. Hospice boards and committees strive to move in two essential directions at once: on the one hand to preserve the autonomy, integrity and flexibility of the hospice team within the health-care establishment; and, on the other hand, to make sure that there is adequate representation from hospital administrations, influential physicians and nurses, and other health-care professionals to ensure that the program will have the attention and support of the medical community. For example, the committee which is responsible for the hospice program at St. Luke's includes the hospital's vice-president for operations, a former president of the board of trustees, a physician currently on the hospital board, the hospital's chief of radiation therapy, the vice-president of the medical board, the hospital's research administrator, the home-care administrator, the director of nursing services, and so on. In other words, teamwork in administration at the top level is as essential as teamwork among the persons actually working with the terminally ill, if the objectives are to be accomplished.

Criteria for Admission

A hospice team cannot work with all those who might apply for help. The New Haven Hospice defines eligibility with three criteria: 1) the patient must have cancer, 2) it must be determined that he or she has only weeks or months to live—rather than years, and 3) the patient/family must reside within the geographical area the hospice is able to serve, 4) consent and cooperation of the patient's own physician must be obtained, and 5) it is preferred that a primary care person be in the home, usually a relative. At St. Luke's Hospital the hospice team may become aware of a patient who is dying and who ought to be involved with the team's ministry, but the patient's physician must first of all be willing for the hospice team to become involved before the team can act in the case. Some physicians are only too ready to get rid of a patient they can not cure, while others may be slow in releasing a patient to the hospice team that it will be too late for anything effective to be done. In addition to the physician's permission, the patient and family must also be willing to participate. The hospice team which works in a hospital has some advantages at this point, in that they can become visible to the family and patient who are considering involvement. A hospice nurse or chaplain can even take a modest initiative by saying, for example: "We are here to help patients like you as much as we can." The St. Luke's team not only limits its patients to those who are suffering from a malignant condition which is in an advanced stage, but preference is given to patients whose symptoms are not being controlled. As of 1976 the team had to limit itself to cancer patients, but recognized that in time the team ought to work with heart disease and diabetes patients also. The physician who is medical director of the hospice team decides if exceptions are to be made and has the final say over which terminally-ill patients are accepted.

By policy, the members of the St. Luke's team are authorized to make rounds of the hospital with floor staff to look for persons who ought to be considered for the hospice program. Such explorations are usually made by a social worker, a nurse from home care, and the nurse who heads the hospice team. Patients they find who meet the criteria for admission to the hospice program are then referred to the hospice medical director for his opinion. After he evaluates the patient's eligibility, he or the clinical specialist (nurse) then approaches the physician in charge to inquire whether or not the hospice team will be invited to become involved in care of the patient. If the physician, patient and his family all concur, then the nurse who heads the hospice team notifies the team members, and they begin to work with members of the hospital staff on that patient's floor, checking the patient on a regular schedule or more often as needed.

Services Provided

At Royal Victoria Hospital, regardless of whether the patient who comes to the Palliative Care Unit is transferred from else where in the hospital or is admitted from home, the goals of admission procedure are the same—to give the patient a sense of reassurance from the very start. The patient is personally welcomed by the nurse who will be in charge, a welcome card with his or her name—and flowers—are on the bedside table. The family and patient are not kept waiting, and any problems —such as any symptoms that need immediate management— are promptly cared for so that the patient is made comfortable. Many patients have arrived with the words ringing in their ears: "*Nothing more can be done in your case.*" The hospice team's reassurance therefore begins by demonstrating that there is a great deal that can be done, starting with excellent symptom control. Strength can be increased to replace weakness; quality of food, along with appetite, can be improved; breathlessness can be alleviated; thirst can be satisfied, and many other discomforts can be handled, such as dry mouth, constipation, bedsores, nausea, diarrhoea, depression, and so on. Then new friends and interests can be provided. Excellent nursing is basic regardless of whether concern is for the physical needs of the patient or the psychological needs of patient or family. The various elements are roughly the same, however, whether the terminally-ill patient is in a facility or is being aided by a hospice team at home. The New Haven Hospice describes its service as including:

—physician consultation on palliative care,
—regular nursing care on call at home seven days a week and 24-hours-a-day, but not private duty nursing,
—social work assistance and consultation, with counseling provided as needed,
—pastoral care consultation as needed through liaison service of the hospice staff to local clergy,
—volunteers to assist as friendly visitors or to help with shopping, transportation, and so on,
—bereavement follow-up as indicated.

Team Co-ordination

At the heart of a hospice program is a weekly meeting of members of the team to discuss and give special consideration to the needs of each individual patient. At St. Luke's, for example, each patient is discussed point by point so that the members of the team will know everything that is going on and thus make sure that what each says or does fits in with the total pattern and plan. Decisions are made as to which member of the team will ask which questions so that they do not duplicate one another's conversation. At the weekly team meetings, the hospital staff is discussed as well as the patients, so that the team can be alerted to staff needs and ways they can be assisted. Such regular discussions also keep members of the hospice team alerted to possible conflicts, so that tensions can be resolved before they become serious. Team meetings also serve to build the relationship among members of the hospice group themselves, so that they can better support one another. They talk things through, plan parties and celebrations together, seek to develop a philosophy of teamwork, and are alert to call on the assistance of a psychiatrist if there is a "blowup."

At Royal Victoria Hospital it was said: "Fundamental to the team approach is the concept that no one person has all the answers and that total care is made easier by a variety of personnel, with a variety of resources, working together. Such a team approach, however, is not an easy task, and members must resolve to break down interprofessional rivalries and set aside defensive attitudes. Communication is essential and requires both time and effort." [3] Good communication is not only verbal through regular meetings but also requires careful records which can be shared. Through co-ordinated records of physicians, nurses, and others, the story of each patient unfolds so as to involve all members of the team. A basic step is *assessment*, recognizing that each family and patient are unique. Members of the hospice team are differing personalities also, with their own ideas about methods of work, their own points of view which may not always be initially in harmony. Especially at the beginning stages of a new hospice program, but also on a continuing basis, the team and administrator must be in dialog and agreement about the job description of each team member. The most helpful way, therefore, to describe a hospice program is to review the tasks and roles of each member of the team.

Team Responsibility: The Physician

Initially, the responsibilities of physicians on a hospice team seem simple and clear. At St. Luke's, for example, after clearing with a patient's physician that the patient is to be permitted in the hospice program and is indeed eligible, the medical director must then take initiative to propose a plan of care. He personally sees each patient once a week, or more often as necessary. He meets with the hospice team to discuss and review the plan of care. He functions as a consultant with any other physician who may be involved either in this specific case or in seeking to be helpful to the hospital staff as a whole. He gives advice to other physicians who request opinions—in managing symptoms of advanced cancer, for example—and he assists in the writing of research proposals and in evaluating the work of the hospice team along with other members.

Must the chairman of a hospice team always be a physician? Not at St. Luke's, where a nurse chairs the team. In some other situations it is proposed that team chairmanship should rotate, so that every major member of the team takes a turn at being team chairman for a period of time. The point of who is actual chairperson becomes unimportant, however, if the team works though all controversies to a point of consensus, and avoids letting physicians rule dogmatically because of their expertise and authority.

The job description and role of hospice physicians will vary considerably from one style of program to another—a fact which, if not noted, could result in some confusion or difficulty. If a hospice patient is at home, for example, the physician may be less necessary, his role being essentially consultative and secondary, with nurses not only assuming primary responsibility but also making many medical decisions. On the other hand, if there is a hospice facility and the physician is employed as director, then his responsibilities become administrative and at many essential points his role may shift. Is it a wise use of medical resources to divert a physician's time to administrative desk work and paper work? Although the nurses will in most cases play the central role in actual patient care, the physician is more likely to be actively involved in a hospital Palliative Care Unit. The physician may see a patient at home only if the patient takes the initiative to call or if the nurse urges the patient to come to an outpatient clinic to see the physician; whereas in a hospital unit the physician will regularly see a hospice patient on his rounds. A physician may choose to use his authority democratically as a member of the team, but there are points under the law where he alone is finally responsible. He must be prepared to stand behind his diagnosis and his prescriptions. The physician in a hospice program needs to recover a quality of personal ministry to add to his medical skill. "The physician engaged in palliative care requires a wide-ranging set of skills embracing a variety of disciplines," it has been pointed out at Royal Victoria.[4] "He at times must be general physician, surgeon, oncologist, and psychiatrist. The most appropriate training ground would appear to be a sound basis in family practice." Still he also gets involved in research, administration, teaching, consultation on cancer problems, and in supervision of students and trainees. The ability to communicate simply and directly is a badly needed skill, and there must be a commitment to, and hopefully some insight into, teamwork.

The physician's underlying authority is not only legal and a matter of status within the health-care system but also is underlined by society's reimbursement at salary levels far above other members of a hospice team. In the general health-care system a social worker or clergyman with equal training and education may not command a third of the salary that a physician may have. In one hospice situation the chaplain has ten years of schooling above college, two years in internship with clinical pastoral training in a hospital beyond that. His education debts are larger than those of the young doctor with fewer years of training who receives a larger salary for his hospice work. A similar sort of authority status may result from the larger income of the primary physician in a case, in contrast with the physician who is on a hospice salary. Will physicians working with the terminally ill be paid less as a subtle recognition by the health-care system that their work is less important?

The family physician may at times indicate positive support for hospice team and physician by saying something like: "We need you when our job is done." But from the perspective of the hospice team, the primary physician's task is not done. If the hospice patient is in the hospital, his previous physician may continue to see him on daily rounds. Even though primary medical responsibility is no longer his, by continuing as a member of the caring team he will at least be sustaining a personal relationship between two friends: family doctor and patient.

Team Responsibility: The Nurses

Whereas there has been a problem in recruiting physicians for hospice work, a director of nursing has found that a "people-oriented" type of care readily attracts capable nurses. The Palliative Care Unit at Royal Victoria seeks nurses who have had five years of broad-based nursing experience, who have an openness to new ideas and methods, and with an orientation to people rather than to technology. The Unit seeks nurses who have not experienced personal bereavement within one year, who have a stable home life with a variety of outside interests, and who have personal maturity and the ability to work as a team member. At St. Luke's the nurses on the hospice team are all clinical specialists—that is, nurses with master's degrees.

The stated aim for nurses in the St. Luke's hospice team is to translate professional skills and human compassion into positive health care to meet the total individual needs of each patient, including psychosocial and spiritual needs. The objectives of nurses on the team are (a) "to assist patients and their families to spend their remaining time in a manner that is meaningful for them," [5] which requires control of symptoms, and (b) to help staff cope with their own personal reactions to death and to gain expertise in applying professional nursing skills to the care of terminally-ill patients.

At Royal Victoria Hospital the nurses follow a normal three-shift rotation, with the majority of palliative-care nurses working full time, supplemented by part-time persons who bring to their work the asset of being less likely to be physically or emotionally fatigued. When nurses work a fixed shift, it tends to isolate some nurses from staff meetings and team participation, so the team seeks to rotate meetings from shift to shift also. A new nurse is integrated into the life of the Palliative Care Unit in a series of stages, beginning with physical orientation on the first day, followed by study of an orientation manual which outlines the unit's philosophy and method of work. During the first week the new nurse is assigned to work in pair with an experienced nurse, then the next week takes on individual responsibility, and by the fourth week is oriented to medication by a nurse-clinician teacher. By the end of two months a new nurse is able to take charge of an evening shift, and a month later can be in charge on a week end with a senior nurse. The patient load, which is 5.5 hours per patient in other departments of the hospital, is 8.5 hours per patient in the Palliative Care Unit in order to provide more time for personal conversation and care.

The specific responsibilities of nursing members in the St. Luke's team include:

—direct care of hospice patients and families,

—collaboration with other disciplines within the hospital and community to co-ordinate care given to patients,

—development and utilization of teaching aides, publications and seminars for the education of staff and volunteers,

—acting as consultants to colleagues, allied personnel, and patients and families,

—promoting and utilizing research which relates to care of the terminally ill,

—developing expertise in the control of prevalent symptoms.[6]

The role of the nurse in the health-care system is gradually being redefined. Nurses not only carry out the orders of doctors but at times—as mediators between physicians and patients—they may take initiative on their own, which may put a strain on the nurse's conscience. But nurses, like patients and families, seem to be seeking less oppressive ways of carrying out their duties. Some of the problems are apparently resolved by the functioning teamwork in hospice programs, which enables nurses to argue more openly for their point of view, and provides a setting within which physicians are better able to hear nurses and work as colleagues with them. One hospice physician said: "I find myself trusting the medical judgment of nurses much more, and even of chaplains who may spend more time with patients than I do. I'm certainly more willing to hear and trust their recommendations." Such respect for nurses is also a function of their continually updated skills and education. At Royal Victoria Hospital, for example, the hospice nurses continually upgrade their expertise through frequent consultation with other team members, through meetings at which each case is reviewed, and through biweekly in-service teaching rounds, as well as through educational programs and conferences which bring specialists from outside into the continuing education program.

A basic skill for a hospice nurse is the ability to listen and to hear. Nurses need to be able to touch a patient gently, warmly, and with compassion, to be thoughtful and competent in emotional concern and care, to be open and willing to seek counsel and help. An ability to listen means being able to know when silence is appropriate also: to be gently honest, not reinforcing denial, when a nurse does speak. "At the same time," an experienced nurse said, "Kübler-Ross's stages of dying must not be taken literally, as always happening in that order. Each person is unique. Young nurses are often tempted to be simplistic in quickly defining a patient's current stage and labeling a comment by a patient as 'bargaining' or 'denial.'" The hospice nurse seeks first of all to develop a personal relationship with a new patient, seeking to help each person in simple ways, by responding to whatever bothers the ill person: "My food is cold" or "Could I have some hot tea?" Or "This sheet is bothering me." One hospice nurse, when asked to specify what is unique about the job description of a nurse on such a team, said: "Nothing you can put on paper. The difference is a spirit, an attitude, something that is contagious, perhaps, rather than learned." Another said: "Good nursing is crucial and requires perceptive evaluation by the nurse herself and by others. In a quest for excellence, we must continually ask what ought to be changed. We must continually discuss with other nurses how skills can be improved and why certain things are done or not done. Critical evaluation is difficult in any situation and especially in a context where there is likely to be some conflict between nurses and physicians, between nurses and head nurse, or among nurses themselves. In the team meetings a nurse can ask for information, can challenge a physician's procedures or judgment, and can openly define her own needs."

The needs of nurses in hospice programs certainly include a lounge to rest in, proper supervision and schedules, as well as adequate salaries. To ignore such personal and basic concerns would be a crucial error. But in many hospitals there is a more serious problem. When a patient dies, attention is given to the grief of the family, but not to the grief of the nurse and her needs at that moment. The death of a young person, for example, close to the age of the nurse, or the death of a child, may be as traumatic for the nurse as for the family—especially if the nurse has worked closely on a personal basis with that patient. Hospital nurses must proceed to wash the body and complete their records as if they have no emotional needs. This is corrected in a hospice unit by sending someone immediately to talk with and work with the bereaved nurse, thus providing her with supportive conversation and help until she is free to go to the nurses' lounge to recover.

"Palliative-care nursing can challenge the skills of any nurse," the Royal Victoria report says.[7] "At the same time it offers great personal satisfactions and rewards if the nurses have time to listen, to understand, and to provide care they can take pride in, which means that the number of nurses, nursing assistants, and orderlies must be adequate for around-the-clock care. The art of caring for the dying is the same as that of all good nursing; what is needed is an acute power of observation, an exquisite sensitivity to the patient's needs, and an infinite capacity for taking pains."[8]

Team Responsibility: Nursing in Home Care

In the hospital the nurse provides basic care. When the patient is at home the role of the hospice nurse shifts radically, as does the role of the physician. At home the family provides basic care, with the nurse as consultant. In addition to skills previously defined, the home-care nurse needs to be able to work independently and takes more individual responsibility, with, of course, the team to back her up. She must carry more of the burden of assessment, defining the complex range of needs a particular patient and family may have, so as to set treatment priorities and limits to intervention. The hospice nurse needs to learn from visiting nurses and community nurses how to co-ordinate care, how to orchestrate other supportive services. The nurse must have patience not only to listen and to understand but also to be able to accept the peculiarities and problems of the patient; not only altered body images and disfigurement of patients but also family limitations and emotional needs. Whatever their deficiencies, patients and families must be treated as adults, regardless of the mothering instincts and habits of a nurse. The nurse may find herself in many non-nursing roles, as she seeks to help members of the family communicate with one another, and puts them in touch with various services to meet non-medical needs.

Team Responsibility: Social Worker

A hospice social worker initially interviews a new patient and family for information which becomes an important part of the team's understanding and records. Illnesses—and terminal sickness more than others—have long been recognized as having financial and social implications. The social worker's training enables him/her to help a family deal with problems such as pensions, wills, and medical bills, as well as implications of death and bereavement. At St. Luke's the social worker begins by asking about:

—the patient's understanding of his or her condition,
—problems raised by terminal illness and their possible solutions,
—the patient's emotional situation—whether anxious, angry, depressed,
—the patient's relationship to family and friends,
—the patient's life-style prior to illness,
—the patient's strengths,

—future plans of the patient and family,

—what special services are needed.

The direct responsibilities of the social worker at Royal Victoria include: (*a*) social assessments, (*b*) case work services, (*c*) placements from home or hospital, (*d*) co-ordination of community services, and (*e*) grief work. The social worker serves as resource person for the hospice team in providing information on community services, *i.e.*, as in relation to home care or for help in managing social problems, and also is involved in research and teaching functions with volunteers, visitors, speaking to outside groups, recommending changes in procedure, and so on. "The social worker, as a team member, provides support to, and receives support from, the team. As a skilled professional, the social worker can serve to guide, reinforce and reassure those less experienced team members who are uncomfortable in areas such as interviewing families, counseling, or dealing with family problems." [9]

In employing a social worker, the Palliative Care Service at Royal Victoria Hospital sought a well-trained professional with:

—three to five years of experience in a hospital or health care setting,

—a master's degree in social work,

—ability to work in a team setting,

—comprehensive knowledge of community resources,

—flexibility to become involved in all aspects of the hospice program if necessary,

—an interest in teaching skills to others as well as in research design and methodology.

Suggested prior training also recommended included conferences or a workshop on care of the dying along with a thorough grounding in grief and bereavement.

Along with chaplains, the social worker can play an important role in some of the most difficult periods a patient faces. If the hospice program is within a hospital, then the social worker's relationship to the social service department of the hospital can make it possible for some help to be provided during the hard time during which it is being decided whether or not to place a particular patient within the hospice program. At Royal Victoria Hospital social workers believe that when a physician delays the decision this is the most difficult time of all for terminally-ill persons.[10] The average time of waiting before placement was actually only 13 days, as compared with an average of 37 days' survival within the Palliative Care Unit.

Some of the varied types of problems a social worker may have to deal with are illustrated by the case of a dying woman whose son had been born with limited eyesight and had been in trouble with the police from the age of fourteen. He was sent to prison for armed robbery, was later paroled, but repeatedly broke his parole. Arrangements were made for the son to visit his terminally-ill mother while under armed guard, but the son escaped and was then sent back for twenty-five years imprisonment without parole. The social worker then had to notify the son in prison about his mother's death.

The social worker frequently needs to assist families with funeral arrangements and in making plans for the care of surviving children or other family members—all of which involves liaison with community social agencies. The social worker also has liaison responsibilities with the patient's physician, floor nurses and aides, and the weekly hospice staff conferences. In most of the hospice programs which were examined, the social worker is assigned major "support functions" for the staff and patient. At St. Luke's, for example, once a patient is sent home the social worker co-operates with the home-care nurses, in making periodic visits to the home and frequent telephone calls to assist the family in securing homemaker assistance or other social agency services. The process is much the same in bereavement work regardless of whether the patient died in the hospital or at home. Royal Victoria's Palliative Care Unit uses a "bereavement coping assessment" instrument and bereavement follow-up checklist which reminds the hospice staff to check on appetite, sleep, weight, human contacts, moods, feelings of guilt, housing, occupation, finances, and so on. The same form for a bereavement visit contact report was used by nurses and social workers.[11]

Team Responsibility: The Chaplain

The New Haven Hospice, working for the most part with patients at home has, not a chaplain, but a pastoral care consultant to seek to work through the patient's own clergyman. At Royal Victoria Hospital, the Palliative Care Unit is dependent upon the hospital's chaplaincy staff, with less specific chaplaincy time assigned to the hospice program than at St. Luke's Hospital. As with other team responsibilities, however, spiritual matters are not delegated to a clergyman and ignored by other members of the hospice team. In addition to the theological education and additional clinical education in a hospital which is recommended for hospital chaplains, the clergy who work as members of a hospice team need to have participated in seminars and training programs on bereavement care and special ministries to the dying. Much more is needed than prayers and last rites, although at Royal Victoria Hospital when daily prayers were added to the program of the Palliative Care Unit, the response of patients and families—as to all aspects of religious ministry—was positive but varied. A woman theological student who participated in and observed the work of the hospice unit was aware that some patients could not accept her religious services because of her sex, and that others were professed atheists or agnostics. Her observations and experience led her to conclude that the most essential functions of religious ministry are listening and talking, moving from there to expressed needs.[12]

Questions of meaning are greatly intensified in any hospital setting, but the religious ministry is limited by attitudes of both patients and staff. Many physicians feel that clergy are a nuisance and should be kept out of the way as much as possible; but a clergyman on the team who can demonstrate his skills and expertise, who can be supportive of members of the staff as well as of patients, can help other clergy with staff problems and help mediate between the medical profession and clergy who lack proper training. The presence of a chaplain on a hospice team helps articulate spiritual problems which otherwise would get only superficial treatment. The director of the Palliative Care Service at Royal Victoria Hospital said that it is not always easy to get spiritual problems to surface. Indeed, it may be that the most serious psychological or religious problems are neglected. The chairman of the board of the New Haven Hospice said: "If a patient shares some strong religious belief with a nurse, or some doubts and concerns, and then asks her to pray with him should she feel obliged to call a chaplain? Or can she be a human being who is willing to share in a personal request and relationship which the patient wants even if all she herself has to do is share in some silence ending with an amen." The St. Luke's policy statement also points out that some other member of a hospice team may be closer to a patient at a given moment than the chaplain and thus can be the one to touch a responsive chord. This illustrates the way staff roles may be blurred in the teamwork process and how each member of a hospice team must be spiritually sensitive. All this requires spiritual support for members of the team. It is one thing to help a person with a warm and healthy faith, and another to try to meet the spiritual needs of someone who is frightened of a God of retribution and eternal punishment. Sometimes members of a hospice staff may need the help of a chaplain in order to deal with a difficult spiritual problem or to meet a request for sacrament.

A chaplain who knows medical language and the milieu of the hospital may be better able to help within the total context of a hospice team than is a parish clergyman called in to deal with occasional problems. A chaplain may also be alert to help a hospice team raise ethical issues that might otherwise be passed over. The chaplain can sometimes mediate conflicts over medical roles, and can often serve as an advocate of the patient and family if they seem to need an ally against medical personnel. Such advocacy may simply be to remind the physicians, in times of pressure, that the helpless patient is still a person and should not be referred to as "that case" or "the vegetable in Room 76." Case studies describing the functioning of a chaplain also underline the chaplain's role in supporting and co-ordinating the team's work with the concerns of parish clergy.

The Patient's Pastor

As was reported previously, at a hospital board hearing for the New Haven Hospice, one member of the board accused the clergy of agitating to establish hospices so they could abdicate their own responsibilities for dying persons. The hospice planners argued quite the contrary: that the hospice worked in close collaboration with parish clergy to provide a context wherein a religious ministry could be more effective, and that all persons who worked with terminally-ill persons were part of a co-ordinated team effort. A spot check of the clergy in the New Haven area, however, reveals one place in which some pastors are indeed glad to be relieved of responsibility. When a pastor discovers a terminally-ill person who is not from his parish—or is related to no other church—or for whom he can do little because the patient is estranged from the church, he is glad to have the hospice staff take over religious responsibilities.

For the most part, however, New Haven clergy report their happiness with the decision of the New Haven Hospice not to have a chaplain—at least until completion of a facility. They agree that basic religious ministry is the responsibility of the patient's own pastor and defined the responsibilities of said pastor to be as follows:

1. He should alert the family to the possibility of hospice care, when it is found to be needed and if the physician has not done so.

2. He should pressure the physician who seems slow or reluctant to investigate the hospice possibility.

3. He should keep in touch with the hospice staff to remind them of clergy interest and availability, and alert the hospice staff to any needs or information the clergyman discovers in his own visits.

4. He should visit the patient and family regularly and make himself available to them in any way they may consider to be helpful, including some initiative in discussing spiritual difficulties and problems.

5. He should inform himself of hospice procedures so that in his own counseling of patient and family he can be supportive of hospice goals and methods.

One pastor said in retrospect: "Perhaps I myself should have sought more guidance from the hospice team, to make sure my counseling was consistent with theirs." Were there any criticisms by clergy of the hospice work and program? One pastor said: "I saw the hospice staff performing a beautiful ministry to a family of my congregation. It was not clear to me, however, just what channels of communication were open between me and the hospice staff, or whether communication from me would be welcome. Perhaps for this reason the hospice needs a chaplain. It was not clear to me whether the hospice staff asked questions of the family about the adequacy of my ministry to them. I am sure my ministry could have been improved through suggestions from the hospice staff." Another pastor said: "If I did not feel needed in the first involvement I had with a hospice family, it was because that husband and wife were spiritually well put together. They had a fine church relationship, were very supportive of each other, and in no sense went to pieces in the crisis. If I did not feel they needed extraordinary attention from me, I think that indicates they didn't need the hospice team as much as some other patients do, either. In the second hospice case where I was involved, the situation was quite different. I saw the hospice people were giving superb care; but, though we did not discuss it, I saw that they were as frustrated as I was about the patient's terrible anxiety over her cancer and impending death. Perhaps it was my function to do more than I did about this anxiety, and maybe I should have consulted more with the hospice staff about this. For when it was over I felt that both the hospice and I had failed to deal adequately with that anxiety. Perhaps it was a failure of skill on my part, and I really don't know if the hospice team could have helped me at the point of my skill weakness."

A priest said: "When the hospice has a facility of its own I am sure I will do a better job working with them. It may be my fault that I am 'place oriented,' accustomed to making hospital calls, for example. Somehow I have a feeling that the hospice staff will be more accessible to me in that place; for, while I feel free to go to people's homes, I am reluctant to approach people in their office unless I am invited. Perhaps there will be a clergy office in the hospice facility, which will help parish clergy to feel that we have a stake and are welcome there."

Another pastor said: "What I saw in that home after the hospice team went to work was a new serenity and confidence on the part of patient and family, the result I think of the simple fact that they now knew where to turn in an emergency. Much anxiety results not from existing problems, but in the worry: What will I do if something happens? Often nothing ever happens that can't be coped with, but I see a great sense of relief when there is this presence of possible help, this channel of communication between patient-family-hospice team. I do think it would have been most helpful to all concerned, however, if I as pastor could at least once have been in the home at the same time they were there. I saw the excellent results of their work, but I never saw *them* in a context in which we could visibly reinforce one another."

Team Responsibility: Psychiatrist

In a hospice program, members of the staff sometimes become depressed—as, for example, when they become heavily involved with a dying person.[13] At Royal Victoria Hospital, therefore, a consultant psychiatrist spends one day a week at the Palliative Care Unit to provide—in this order of priority—supportive help for the staff, for the family, and for the patients. A psychiatrist gives one-fourth of his time to the work of the hospice team at St. Luke's, often ·making rounds with the nurses in order to see patients, especially those reported to be depressed or demanding. The St. Luke's team psychiatrist has regular hours set aside for counseling of family members. He attends a nursing staff conference on Mondays and a hospice team meeting on Tuesdays. He works also with bereaved families as requested. It is his responsibility to help the staff maintain open communications and to provide them support when they have emotional problems.

The members of a hospice team accept responsibility as healers in a richer and broader sense than the physician often defines for himself, just as they accept responsibility for family feelings (bereavement counseling), for example. The emotional burden of working with the dying might be defined by a phrase used by Nouwen: "wounded healers." [14] Nouwen suggests that in American society a person's self-concept and emotional strength is dependent on feedback he receives from others largely in response to his own work. In the midst of grief and death it is not always easy for a hospice team's members to sustain a healthy perspective, or continually to be able to open themselves to the needs of others. Nouwen warns that in most human institutions people are more concerned with *cure*—that is, with solving problems—than with *caring* for persons. Success and approval from outside generally follow *curing*, not *caring*. The crucial problems he sees is that *cure grows out of care*. At the heart of any successful hospice program, therefore, or of any teamwork and help for persons that is authentic and really effective, there must be a strengthening of team members so that they can really care. Many people are unable to care, to allow themselves really to become involved with other persons, because they simply haven't the strength, the room in their lives and emotions for other people. They seek to avoid pain rather than to help persons in pain.

Nouwen, whose reflection combines the pastoral and the psychiatric, says: "Cure without care can be more harmful than helpful. Notice how many cured patients leave hospitals angry and hostile at their doctors. Our best efforts at social reform wound people." Members of a hospice team must find the strength—and this is one of the support functions of the psychiatrist on a team—from each other to be able to participate in suffering, to have the courage to be with people rather than running away, so that through love and concern suffering can be transformed into self-discovery and growth. The physician and others on the team can then continue to *care*, even when they cannot *cure*.

Team Responsibility: Volunteers

A team can train, supervise and support part-time and volunteer workers—thereby greatly increasing possible services—in ways which are not possible when such teamwork is lacking. What do volunteers do in a hospice program? They read to patients, write letters for them, talk and sympathize—which is often most helpful—and they play cards and games, play records, as well as helping with children or other family members.[15] They also run errands, help in the office, do library cataloging, help with fund-raising, make home visits, and provide transportation. At Royal Victoria Hospital the volunteers help with welcoming new patients, shop for patients, pray with patients, take patients on walks, and if a family member cannot do so may be present with a patient at time of death. When a volunteer has a good relationship with a family he or she may help with bereavement work, with volunteers sometimes setting up and running "bereavement evenings." Volunteers can provide many helpful services for hospice staff members, and at Royal Victoria Hospital they organize the monthly staff parties. At St. Luke's they do most of the office work, arrange flowers, and some who are themselves nurses help in more skilled ways. It has been suggested that volunteers should be recruited who have special skills, instead of merely relying on volunteers who may bring their own problems into the situation—for volunteers are accepted to provide care, not to receive it.[16] A so-called "volunteer pledge" suggests that volunteers:

—promise to be punctual and conscientious in carrying out responsibilities,
—keep all information confidential, taking any criticisms to the director of volunteers,
—endeavor to keep their work standards high in order to uphold the quality of a hospice program,
—always work with consideration, courtesy, and dignity.

Volunteers are generally not welcomed to work in a hospice program, however, unless they are willing to be trained. The New Haven Hospice has a director of volunteers, and Royal Victoria Hospital has a "volunteer coordinator" who is part of the Palliative Care Unit's administrative team. She is one of the two interviewers for all prospective volunteers, does a great deal of counseling with volunteers—both in person and on the telephone—and she is responsible for assigning and scheduling the work of volunteers, who generally work once a week on a three- or four-hour shift—for example, 9:00 A.M. to 1:00 P.M., 1:00 P.M. to 5:00 P.M., and 5:00 P.M. to 9:00 P.M. Volunteers are trained through a course which includes films, panel presentations by the hospice staff, and readings. Each spring new volunteers are encouraged to take a course on death and dying at McGill University. In-service training takes place further at monthly meetings of volunteers, which are also occasions for the volunteers to support and help one another. The fifty to sixty volunteers in the Montreal program, often able to work two at each shift, bring varied contributions to the hospice work, often supplying a "freshness and vitality which helps both staff and families."

The New Haven Hospice had forty-six volunteers in 1975, who were oriented through meetings and readings on pain control, the meaning of death, the role of the family, bereavement, and so on. Many volunteers were then assigned as a part of training to travel for a time with a home-care nurse in order to obtain personal experience in helping a nurse with various phases of work. The director of volunteers has said: "Volunteers take a lot of time but they are so valuable as to be worth the investment." One of the ways in which volunteers are recruited is by inviting the public or persons who have inquired to a first Thursday open house at which an audiovisual presentation of hospice work is made, followed by a period in which persons present ask questions of the hospice staff. One volunteer said: "It's rewarding work, with some hard days—but they aren't the times when someone dies. Rather it is the anxiety of patients and families which is most difficult. Or the really difficult problems which no one can deal with adequately. Still, one can listen and hold hands, and that is most valuable at times when problems can't be solved." A director of volunteers said: "One must, of course, take care to match volunteers skills with patient needs carefully; some people hit it off together and others do not."

Team Responsibility: Research

The goals of the initial research at Royal Victoria Hospital were to determine the nature of the emotional and physical needs of terminally-ill persons; the areas of deficiencies in meeting these needs, along with possible means of correcting these deficiencies. The continuing research of the Palliative Care Unit expands upon those fundamental directions. Research areas have included: (a) evaluation policy, (b) demographic data, (c) cost analysis to determine how much money the hospice program saves the hospital, (d) pain study, (e) patient stress study, (f) bereavement follow-up evaluation, (g) impact of stress upon staff, (h) home-care program evaluation, (i) case studies, (j) consumer response, and so on.[17] The patient stress research, for example, sought to develop and test questionnaires for use in measuring the changing levels of stress experienced by patients who died within the palliative-care program, as opposed to those who died outside a hospice program.

While most of the Royal Victoria research has been conventional, the Palliative Care Unit collaborated with the director of research of the New Haven Hospice in a more controversial experiment by using a participant observation technique to find out what was going on in the hospice unit. "Participant observation" is a technique originally developed for anthropological study of native cultures, with the observer living among the subjects he is studying so that he can be intensely and continuously involved with them. Then the procedure was adapted to the study of modern institutions, with a scientist going to prison as a convict in order to study prison culture, and so on. In a similar way the director of research from the New Haven Hospice was aided by colleagues in Montreal to be admitted as a patient dying of cancer of the pancreas. The story of the pseudo-patient's experiences have been reported in the press,[18] and his findings with regard to the quality of care in a surgical ward versus the hospice unit are analyzed in a more scholarly report.[19] He found that patients experienced monotony and loneliness on the surgical ward, while kindness and individual attention were experienced in the hospice unit. His participation did not uncover striking new facts, but did serve to provide more evidence for the value and effectiveness of hospice programs.

Team Responsibility: Public Relations

While research provides sound evidence for certain types of evaluation of hospice programs, some observers worry that hospice programs may fall into the situation of the health-care system in general, which makes inadequate provision for the outside non-medical evaluation of medical programs. Adequate evaluation requires adequate criteria. Are such criteria to be developed within the health-care system without consulting society at large and considering its goals? Certain types of evaluation—such as a psychiatric institute's study of the impact of hospice work on the emotions of hospice staff persons—require perhaps an evaluation from within the medical establishment, but Frank Kryza II, the highly competent and imaginative public relations director of the New Haven Hospice saw that an important way to win the confidence and support of the public and the larger community was to involve a wider range of disciplines in the process of evaluation and criteria setting. Public relations commonly involves press releases, public meetings and documents to interpret the work of a program, along with preparing informative leaflets and reports, but all of these means of building public support and sharing information are more effective if the process of research and evaluation turns out significant information which will challenge the attention of the public.

The New Haven Hospice therefore sought to look at its

work and have it evaluated in a larger context. Where the first thought of many persons planning hospice programs is to ask how a hospice model can help change the entire health-care system, the New Haven Hospice began an experiment of taking an even larger and more comprehensive approach: looking at the hospice program and the needs of the terminally ill in the context of the deepest problems of contemporary society, while at the same time avoiding two dangers: that of professional people evaluating themselves on one hand, and that of concentrating research and evaluation on very small and manageable projects on the other. A grant was obtained from the Connecticut Humanities Council to establish a panel of experts from the humanities—not directly from medical science—who would be involved in a series of symposia addressed to the general community of science and learning asking fundamental evaluative questions more basic than the establishment of criteria for evaluation itself. For example, the first of the symposia, held on November 22, 1976 in New Haven, addressed itself to the question of "Dying and the Media," with an in-depth analysis of the problem of death in a bureaucratic society. The experiment will be closely watched for its impact upon the hospice movement, and as perhaps establishing a means and precedent for another type of evaluation of health-care programs. The initial discussions in 1976 were highly significant in the way they illuminated basic hospice concepts and needs with perspectives from literature, television, films, and a variety of other suggestive devices.

On one hand, "It is difficult if not impossible to measure the impact of caring, a decrease in isolation, an increase in communication, a decrease in loneliness" and other aspects of hospice care.[20] On the other hand, a medical-school professor who did not wish to be named said: "It is a myth that only physicians can evaluate physicians. The medical profession needs to grow up and recognize the larger community's stake in evaluating and improving its services, which means at least one outsider, at least one person from another profession or discipline, to match every doctor involved in evaluating a medical plan, institution, service or program like the hospice." Another observer said: "While I cannot prove it, I am convinced that those persons assigned by the National Cancer Institute to evaluate programs such as a hospice, are oriented toward a kind of research that has a negative impact not only on the type of research a hospice will undertake but also has a subtle effect upon the nature of the hospice program—in negative ways. For example: are any of the persons involved in evaluating grant proposals involved in active patient care? And not only should we ask about their active involvement in Oncology but also whether their concerns are human and personal, whether their criteria for evaluation lead the hospice researchers down the typical research path of depersonalized statistics and attempts to measure pain levels or whatever. Personally I feel that doctors are the only ones qualified to evaluate the work of doctors, but if we are the only ones who can answer the questions, then ways must be found to make sure that society at large—and the consumers of medical care—at least have more of a chance to ask the questions." It is significant that the evaluation-research in the extensive documentation at the Royal Victoria Palliative Care Unit relies so heavily on case studies, and upon recorded "soft evaluation by the consumer, the patient and family" which "may be more meaningful and significant than hard evaluation attempting to determine the statistical significance of some induced change." [21]

Bereavement Evaluation

At Royal Victoria Hospital the study of bereavement and the impact of the hospice program upon it centered around the family member identified as the key person. A pre-bereavement assessment form was used to determine which persons were most likely to be at risk during bereavement. Then one full-time nurse on the hospice staff was assigned as "bereavement follow-up nurse" for a month at a time. This nurse was responsible for a Palliative Care Unit chart for each patient and the recording of all contacts by staff with the patient and family. A phone call was made to the key person two weeks following the death, a home visit was made one month after the death, and a six-month questionnaire was sent to the key person later. A one-year questionnaire followed, along with an anniversary card sent to the key person. Meanwhile a weekly bereavement meeting with psychiatrist, social worker and nurses attempted to review each case to determine which key persons required additional help and to arrange follow-up. Despite some initial difficulties the system worked and even improved with experience. Two wine and cheese evenings were held at the hospital for all key persons at which they were given a chance to express their feelings and tell about their experiences.

Team Responsibility: Training

While the personnel varies from team to team, other important persons commonly involved in hospice care include: 1) a physiotherapist who seeks to relieve discomfort of patients, 2) a pharmacologist, 3) a laboratory technician, 4) a dentist, 5) an occupational therapist, 6) a dietician, and possibly others. An effort is made to help all of these persons to catch the hospice spirit so that they can be helpful and positive in all of their relationships. Many such persons can be involved in training programs such as are conducted by the New Haven Hospice for nursing associations, community agencies, religious groups. It is not easy for a new program like this to develop its own staff and to meet local training needs, while at the same time assisting health-care workers clear across the continent. National conferences for hospice staffs and others interested have nevertheless been conducted in New Haven and Montreal, and there are continuing education programs at St. Luke's. The New Haven Hospice proposes to develop further training programs for health-care professionals for teaching principles and theory—with concurrent clinical experiences—to enable participants to observe the application of principles in practice. The specific educational aims of such a training program—including the continuing education and refresher courses to be held in the future, include:

—exploring the learner's feelings concerning cancer, altered body image, pain, loss, dying, the dying patient, so that the learner can be helped to recognize and deal with these feelings before attempting to assist a dying patient/family,

—developing an attitude of hopefulness that can be transmitted to those receiving care,

—alleviating patient discomfort through sensitivity to the family unit,

—developing collaborative skills to ensure the full benefit of multidisciplinary and volunteer involvement in a comprehensive patient-care program,

—applying adult education principles in teaching self-care to patients and their families,

—establishing realistic limitations for one's own performance in order to assure a staff member's recognition of the need for periodic refreshment.

FOR FURTHER READING

On bereavement, see Clayton, P. J., "Mortality and Morbidity in the First Years of Widowhood," *Arch. Gen. Psychiat.*, 1974, 30; Parkes, C. M. *et al. The First Year of Bereavement.* New York: John Wiley and Sons, 1974; Vachon, M., "Nurses Can Help the Bereaved," *Canadian Nurse*, January 1975; Vachon M. *et al.*, "Stress Reaction to Bereavement," *Essence*, 1976, 1, p. 23. "Bereavement Follow-Up, July–Aug, 1975," in *1976 Report, Royal Victoria, op. cit.*, pp 370 ff; Powledge, T. M., "Death as an Acceptable Subject," *New York Times*, July 25, 1976.

8

Advice to Other Communities

From its inception the New Haven Hospice has sought to give counsel—through publications, consultation, personal conversation—to persons wishing to explore the possibility of a hospice program in their community because from its inception and in its requests for funding the New Haven Hospice has stated its purpose to be a national demonstration center for experimentation which can be shared across the continent. What advice from the limited experience of existing American hospices can be offered to the stream of visitors who come to New Haven?

A Steering Committee with Vision

A significant new type of institution or program does not come into existence unless several people get a vision of its possibility and are excited enough to work long hours as volunteers with enthusiasm so as to make their vision contagious enough to enlist others. The hospice vision includes a feeling of compassion for dying persons and their families, as well as demonstrable evidence that terminally-ill persons can be made more comfortable and happier. Generally speaking, this vision will have little impact upon a community, however, until some study is made of the need and of the existing situation. How many terminally-ill people are there in the area to be served? Are they mainly in institutions or at home? Such information gathered for hospices elsewhere will suggest the questions to be asked.

In the process of making such an initial survey a preliminary planning group or steering committee is generally formed, and its second task may well be to prepare a carefully written statement of alternatives for meeting the need which is being described. At this stage it would probably be unwise for the nature of the proposed program to be prescribed. For example, while some persons are always interested in constructing a new building, a hospice program may be developed within an existing facility. Initially, alternatives should be described in a way that will ask questions and involve as many people as possible in the decision. A larger, more representative planning group is needed for the step-by-step planning which should precede specific proposals and in the negotiations with various health-care agencies and community organizations which should be involved in hospice planning. The people who serve on this larger planning group, as well as the steering committee, need vision and enthusiasm, but there is more. Key health-care people and members of the community's power structure must be included. Success is more likely if nurses and physicians are closely involved, as well as clergy, business people, an attorney, and persons with skill and an insight into organization and fund raising.

It would be a major mistake if the key persons involved in leadership for a proposed hospice organization were known to be critical of the medical establishment in the community, without persons from health-care structures being present equally. One strategy which has been recommended is to send a representative cross-section group to visit an existing hospice program. When they return they can help interpret slides and films of hospice programs at a large community meeting, set up to include official representation from all organizations that ought to be interested and involved, not overlooking representatives of hospitals and nursing homes. Anyone who might later be critical or have influence in blocking the project should know that he or she was invited at this early stage to have a hand in developing the idea and its point of view. At the same time caution should be taken that the newspapers—with the enthusiasm they may have for a new idea—do not build up false impressions in the community. News stories can easily stress sensational or wrong aspects with, for example, headlines stating that a new type of hospital is 'being planned which will be competitive to existing hospitals, or they may sensationally stress the hospice as a program to help people die rather than helping them live until they die.

Initial Research

Sooner or later, choices must be made between alternatives. Should a hospice team be developed within a local hospital? Should space be leased within a nursing home or hospital for a hospice experiment? Careful study and research by competent individuals is needed to secure the essential information for discussion, evaluation, and implementation by the planning group. Two separate kinds of research may be needed: *Medical research* on pain control and other aspects of the existing care for terminally-ill persons may be undertaken by health-care professionals. *Policy research,* collecting facts and figures for community decision, may begin with a study of administrative and program matters, financial possibilities, interagency agreements, legal questions, planning procedures. Should someone with hospice expertise and experience be employed to shape the program and organization, as in New Haven? Or should the community first determine what is needed locally and then employ staff who are committed to that approach?

Careful research and continuing evaluation are essenital

for securing and continuing financial grants from foundations and government sources. It is in any case important to build sound research and evaluation procedures into the structure of any new community organization or service. The director of research at New Haven Hospice urges that clearly defined goals and objectives be formulated as the first essential step in demonstrating the legitimacy, the effectiveness, and the value of a hospice operation. Responsible evaluation will then seek to determine the extent to which these goals are being accomplished, and what program changes or improvements are necessary. It is necessary to examine *structure*, which includes point of view, resources available, population to be served; *process*, which includes describing and analyzing procedures and services; and *outcome*, which seeks a testable design for evaluating the goal to be accomplished.

Building a Power Base

The persons who were studying the project of creating a hospice program in New Haven organized, at an early stage, a series of task forces as a means of enlisting more people in the initial study and planning even while it was still in the idea stage. These task forces, organized to deal thoroughly with one phase of the work of the potential organization, were a means for approaching large numbers of influential persons in order to get them involved. Key people in health care, the business community, and government could thus be involved in the planning from the beginning. Some of these persons continued their involvement into later organizational work, still others "talked up" the hospice idea and enlisted the interest of other persons.

A second means for preparing the community for a careful consideration of the hospice concept was to approach influential organizations and ask them to endorse the idea officially. In order for the boards of directors of these community agencies and institutions to responsibly act on such a request it was necessary for them to inform themselves thoroughly about the hospice idea. This, in turn, gave members of the hospice planning group the opportunity to present their idea and documentation to many such key groups, and to discuss the idea at sufficient length to discover which members of these boards were the most interested and which were least interested in the hospice idea. Those who were found to be quite interested provided a reservoir of potential leadership for fund raising and public relations. They could be approached again for suggestions on ways to enlist the interest and support of their more reluctant colleagues. The reasons why some were not interested provided insights into problems to be studied, data to be gathered, and proposals to be reshaped. Such organizational endorsements were secured, for example, from the boards of directors of all the hospitals in the New Haven area; from regional church agencies and local congregations; from regional and local associations of nurses and agencies like the Visiting Nurses Association; from boards of directors of nonprofit nursing homes and homes for the elderly; from agencies such as the Jewish Family Services, the Junior League, the Mental Health Association, the Rehabilitation Center, and from the faculties of nearby medical schools and schools of health, and so on. The various agencies listed here suggest the scope of endorsements which can be sought in another community. Each community, however, should have its own strategy for determining the politic order of seeking such endorsements. One might, for example, begin first with those agencies which are almost certain to endorse the hospice idea, in the hope of creating a steamroller effect in which agencies which might initially have been reluctant to endorse would be impressed by the impressive list of endorsements already secured.

Actual collaborative relationships are, of course, more important than endorsements. It is, on the one hand, essential to pay close attention to areas of resistance from other agencies that fear a hospice program as potentially competitive, or as possibly overlapping and interfering with their work. Rather than seeking to "sell" such agencies on the virtues of the hospice concept, the officers of related and similar programs must be consulted and in many cases invited to negotiate a possible basis for collaboration. The amount of initial resistance encountered in the New Haven community and from health-care agencies should not be minimized. Some agencies simply viewed the hospice as unnecessary, as duplicating programs already in existence. Other agencies, even though they were more perceptive of the fact that in many cases terminally-ill persons were not being properly cared for, saw the hospice program as a competitor for limited funds they preferred to see used for their own work.

Some of the success of the New Haven Hospice is therefore due to the collaborative relationships which were negotiated with such agencies as the Community Health Center Plan (provides comprehensive preventive health care and other medical services for a large population from labor unions), Connecticut Regional Medical Program, the South Central Connecticut Comprehensive Health Planning Board of Directors, the New Haven unit of the American Cancer Society and its Service and Rehabilitation Committee, the Connecticut Mental Health Center, the Regional Visiting Nurse Associations in New Haven and seven adjacent communities; the Veterans Administration Hospital and all other hospitals, Yale University Divinity School, as well as the Yale School of Medicine, School of Nursing, Health Services, and Yale-New Haven Hospital's Committee on the Role of the Hospital in Addressing Community Health Needs. Such a list suggests the vast amount of work and the complicated web of interrelationships which had to be established or untangled, as the case might be, as well as the variety of supportive and collaborative services which were available.

While the hospice concept is in a sense a response to some

failure not merely of the health-care system but of our entire society in its approach to death and dying, its approach to such agencies could not be negative and critical. There had to be the recognition that many good deaths take place in hospitals, however a "good death" may be defined. What was needed in the community was collaboration among good agencies and services, so that their combined effect could be greatly improved.

Pilot Funds and Funding

As will be discussed in the next chapter, hospices are a feasible innovation in American communities only if they can be funded in the long run through public and private insurance reimbursements for individual patients. However, many communities have local foundations which will provide "seed money" for the initial and exploratory work of a significant new program, but only if there are realistic long-term plans. If a hospice facility is to be constructed or equipped, large amounts of money may have to be raised from location contributions, which means that hardheaded business leaders must be involved in the planning from the very earliest stages. A next step, therefore, is to incorporate a legally constituted hospice agency with officers and a board of directors authorized to solicit and receive funds. Even if the option of a hospice program within a local hospital is being seriously considered, there are many reasons to still proceed with the incorporation of a hospice institution so as to negotiate the arrangement and program on community terms rather than on the basis most advantageous and convenient to a hospital.

Once a board is incorporated, it can solicit funds from foundations and individuals to employ initial staff, perhaps on a part-time basis. Or at least funds can be found for the expenses of volunteers who can write grant proposals, prepare interpretative material, and establish an organization for facilitating the next steps. Once there is an incorporated agency, it is in a position to work out written agreements with co-operating agencies and health-care officials. Not only can future conflict be better avoided and resolved on the basis of written agreements, but clarity and precision of thought is stimulated by the discussion of such documents as are necessary to define the goals, program, services, and relationship to other agencies of the proposed hospice program; as well as what is expected from other agencies by way of services, information, and co-operation.

Even when a new agency or hospice institution is not being created, it has been found helpful to secure written agreements with various departments and divisions of a hospital where a hospice program may be located in order to make sure there is a clear understanding of what is involved from all persons and groups that may be related. Sometimes such agreements may require hours of negotiation as potential problem areas are debated point by point. Legal contracts may be necessary with some community agencies that are expected to provide services; as, for example, with a public health agency or Visiting Nurse Association. With such advance work completed, it is then possible for volunteers to secure grants from foundations or perhaps even from the National Cancer Institute or from some other state or local government agency. St. Luke's Hospital, for example, received an initial $60,000 grant for its hospice experiment from the national women's organization of the Episcopal Church, and in New Haven, Congregational and Episcopal churches loaned $69,500 from permament funds.

Criticisms of the Hospice Concept

Rather than becoming defensive about criticism, which is especially a possibility when a group with vision feels it is being opposed by persons who have no idea what is really being proposed, each criticism can be used as an opportunity for further study, clarification, and interpretation to the community. No idea is perfect, so there are legitimate objections to hospices and worries about how they may develop. Is there a danger that the hospice facility will become just another elitist service for the well-to-do, without any provision for the poor? Will the health-care establishment relax its growing concern for the terminally ill with the assumption that hospices will solve the problem for them, so that changes will not be needed elsewhere in the system? Is the hospice idea encouraging overspecialization and the danger that death will become another specialty, further fragmenting the health-care system?

Some physicians feel that the hospice movement is not adequately prepared for its extreme vulnerability to attack in the long run—an attack which may not be direct, but, instead, a subtle erosion by neglect and uninterest on the part of influential health-care leaders. The hospice movement must operate with a sense of trust, in accordance with the virtues of compassion, prudence, justice, and at times heroism, living by faith in an age which often seems faithless. Hospice staff respect death in a time when death is viewed as a problem to be solved and not as a mystery to be held in awe. In fact, one medical school professor said in confidence, those who hope science can defeat death will not give up their opposition to the hospice notion that dying people should be removed from heroic measures and scientific experimentation so that they can enjoy life at the end. Such medical researches may be silent in the face of the hospice movement at the moment of its popularity and research findings which show the limitations and failures of the health-care system in serving the terminally ill at present, but they will persist in perhaps unvoiced opposition. They will attack the hospice idea whenever they can at the points of its weakness—that is, its compassion and trust. There is no evidence that our society really wants to spend large sums on compassion—whether in caring for children or juvenile deliquents, or the aged . . . or the dying. Cancer money is designed for research to cure cancer, and the hospice people must not be allowed the illusion that it is going to be easy to change the direction of the whole health-care system with its passion for cure, for paying attention to the disease rather than to the person.

A physician in a hospital with a hospice program said: "Despite all of our official administrative support, the hospice team members must recognize that we are in hostile territory. We are fighting rules at every point, and we are competing for funds that influential people want to use for technology and cure." There is not much precedence within American society at present to give encouragement to the hope that a concept like the hospice can win its way without a battle. The problem, as Professor David Stannard of Yale pointed out in a symposium sponsored by New Haven Hospice, is not deficiencies in the health-care system but in our entire bureaucratic, depersonalized, cynical society. "We have shifted from a moral to a technological order," he suggested, "and the evidence that compassionate institutions can survive with integrity is not present in the experience of day-care centers, nursing homes, and other institutions that have had a such a vision in their inception. Most of us," Stannard said, "will die in a ritually organized bureaucratic institution where life dribbles out, where nurses complain that people take so long to die, and where every effort is made to keep a patient alive until the next shift by any heroic measures necessary so as to let someone else take the blame for the failure which death in the hospital represents."

Convincing the Doubters

Holden quotes critics who "warn that no scientific evaluation has been made of hospice care and that evidence of success is largely anecdotal." [1] He cautions that the zeal of certain hospice advocates has the effect of turning off some physicians who might otherwise be interested. Perhaps a majority of health-care professionals are still convinced that they can solve the problem with a few minor changes in the system. A number of skeptics have been convinced by visits to St. Christopher's Hospice in London, or to New Haven or Montreal hospice, but convincing the doubters and answering the critics in a community exploring the idea of establishing a hospice may require more than that. Influential health-care personnel may not finally be persuaded until they have had personal experience with patients of their own in a hospice-like experiment. Medical persons are generally convinced by demonstration rather than by argument.

A hospice program therefore may need to evolve gradually in most communities, as more and more people discover the new possibilities for treatment of dying persons. Certainly most smaller communities could not in any case develop a hospice facility such as is planned in New Haven, or even such as the plan in Washington, D.C.—in connection with the Vince Lombardi Cancer Center—to remodel a floor of the Washington Home for Incurables to make it available for twenty-five terminal cancer patients. Even larger communities cannot expect a hospice program to appear in full bloom and ready to function. "A hospice program begins at the bedside of dying patients, with realistic efforts to assess their needs and possibilities," a nurse says. The clergy may be enlisted as allies in many situations, but it is important that from the beginning persons in each community should know their limitations. Instead of beginning with a vision, many people can begin by asking questions about specific cases and persons as the most effective way to involve nurses and physicians in new possibilities. Practical experience in specific cases may also be influential with local persons or foundations that can provide seed money. The New Haven Hospice, for example, was able to say in several funding requests: "*After three years of work with patients in existing health facilities*, we conclude that there is a need for a health delivery system to help patients round out their lives and live with meaning even though they are dying of degenerative irreversible disease" [italics added]. On the basis of such concrete experience, with data collected by chaplains, nurses, and physicians, that group was able also to point to significant financial savings for the community—less money would be needed from families, hospitals, government, insurance companies—if a hospice program were established.

Legal Questions

Legal counsel will be required to work carefully through laws and regulations of a specific community and state in relation to a variety of legal hurdles which can be anticipated and others which may be raised unexpectedly. A new institution must prepare itself to avoid lawsuits and legal challenges wherever possible. What, for example, are the insurance liabilities for staff and facilities? When lethal dosages of drugs are turned over to families for home-care administration is anyone liable if an accidental death occurs? [2] Is a negligence or malpractice suit a danger if some family or disgruntled employee decides that drugs are being improperly used? Those who make decisions about terminally-ill people must be as careful as those who work in other medical areas, because there are always lawyers and families interested in making money from a lawsuit. Is a hospice liable to a lawsuit if a dying youngster with leukemia is permitted to go home for a few happy days with his family although he might have lived a bit longer had he stayed in the hospital under intensive care?

A new range of legal issues is presented which are not covered by current efforts to make state laws more precise about the nature of death; although it is perhaps implicit in the hospice philosophy that living involves *personality* and *consciousness* and not merely *body functioning*. In 1976 the

state of California passed a "Natural Death Act," the implications of which will be of great interest to persons considering
a hospice program. This act includes a special set of clauses
dealing with persons in extended-care facilities, and represents
a first, preliminary, effort by one state to deal with dying and
the right to die. Death *can* be defined, whereas it may be most
difficult to define *dying* and to deal with it legally. The law
must speak for others who might in the future be influenced by
precedents; also, the rights of the sick, of patients in institutions,
involve many unresolved legal issues. (Reimbursement law is
discussed in the next chapter.)

Specially Trained Staff

A community could construct a hospice facility after a successful campaign had raised millions of dollars, and could secure a
budget of hundreds of thousands of dollars to operate a hospice
program, and still fail to implement the hospice philosophy and
program if the right staff persons could not be found. For example, it is essential from the beginning to have the services of
a physician who is committed to palliative care for dying persons and who is skilled and well informed in pain care. That
physician, in turn, must have the co-operation of a pharmacologist who is able and willing to prepare the prescribed combinations of narcotics. There must be at least a few nurses, a
social worker, some clergy, and other persons—all of whom
are prepared to help implement the hospice objectives. Especially will be needed skilled, experienced, and committed
nurses. Additional staff can be recruited and trained once a
few skilled and perceptive persons are at work demonstrating
what can and should be done for the terminally ill. However
useful other hospice programs may be as places for training
and demonstration—and new staff from many communities
will no doubt be sent to the hospice for this purpose—each
new hospice program must develop a team of skilled persons
who will educate one another with a process of team- and self-

education built into the process. No one is adequately qualified for hospice work, so well-qualified persons are those who are prepared to continue growing and learning, changing in response to the need and the situation, which is a continual learning laboratory for them if they share and interpret together what they are learning from their actual work with dying persons.

In most communities the right staff will not be found ready trained, clearly perceptive, and sensitive to the hospice point of view. People with a commitment and a "feel for it" can be trained, however; and, in time, centers like New Haven Hospice will perhaps develop a new type of certified training, with clinical instruction and interneships. Even so, it may well be that a certain type of personality is required, the sort of person who is not too busy and fragmented to be able to enter sensitively into the lives of others. Where does one look for such a person? Such wholeness is not easily come by in the life of a physician or specialized nurse—in part because of the pressure engendered by the very process of education. The hospice nurses at St. Luke's Hospital seek to recover the needed wholeness and human perspective through Bible study together; other hospices do this through efforts at nurturing teamwork.

Team Building

In every area of modern life as knowledge expands and becomes more specialized, and as technology and organization become more complex, the issue of teamwork becomes increasingly important. Early teamwork in medicine was largely based upon an authoritarian model, and as that model withers away in interdisciplinary work, a team may find itself like a troika with each horse pulling in a conflicting direction. As traditional roles blur into a mingling of expertise and skills, the question of who has authority no longer matters, giving way instead to enabling roles, with leadership passed from one member of a team to another, depending on which member has the skill or the enabling function needed at the time. Team skills include the ability to resolve conflict, to bring out the voice and contribution of each team member, as well as the skill of enabling an authoritarian team member to become less paternalistic and more open to the sense and will of the group.

Planners of a new hospice may want to explore T-group and sensitivity training methods helpful in developing teamwork, but there are structural suggestions which may also be helpful, adapted from the experience of teamwork in other areas: team teaching, clergy teams, teams in business. Teamwork, as a process by which persons learn to work together effectively by building and maintaining a spirit of trust and collaboration, is hard work. Just as a person's health deteriorates if neglected, so also does the health of team functioning. Team members must feel free to state openly their hopes and fears about the team tasks. They must receive recognition for their skills, and support for their deficiencies. A basic question at each meeting is: What are we learning about each other and what are we doing? Team skills include the ability to bring conflict out into the open and to deal with it. This is not to say that tensions are easily resolved, but they can be the occasion for identifying political involvements, for clarifying role definitions and job descriptions, as well as present ways of working that hinder teamwork. The notion that there can be an ideal team is a myth, because highly motivated and skilled persons will inevitably come to some fundamental disagreements. The more visionary the goals, the more idealistic the program, the more likely its excellent theory will come into conflict with the habitual styles of staff work and personalities. Ingrained individualism and professional perogatives do not easily yield to a style of work which puts the good of others—the patients and other team members—ahead of personal preferences.

The most difficult tensions in teams may be when personalities clash, especially when a program involves the sort of creative professional persons who are most likely to be drawn to an innovative, experimental project. Creative people can be temperamental in demanding their own way, and the people most verbally committed to a philosophy or way of work may shift ground when budget priorities become crucial. Compassionate people may be unwilling to deal promptly and competently with the laziness or incompetence of persons with whom they have developed personal team relations. A team enabler who keeps records of all agreements, who reminds each team member of responsibilities and assignments, who sees that committees function and that evaluations are made on time, can help at keeping problems on the surface, but is dependent upon written agreements and assignments. A British hospice physician said that "as long as the patient's welfare is considered first a team spirit will arise naturally." American hospice experience, on the other hand, suggests that this is by no means so inevitable, but requires careful planning from the beginning as well as attention to the enabling skills that are required. Initially the teamwork at New Haven Hospice was developed through socials and frequent meetings. In the plans for the Palliative Care Unit at Royal Victoria Hospital, attention was given in each area of team functioning to provide for team and, when necessary, psychiatric support for the individual, and psychiatric support for the team—to make sure, for example, that teamwork was not disabled by personal stress or problems.

It is inevitable that regular team meetings at a hospice will at times become emotional, and that staff members may find it easy to neglect crucial issues or meetings in order to avoid emotion. There are persons engaged in hospice programs, or in planning them, who would minimize the importance of team building as a process. They resent the necessity of clearing everything with many people, and would prefer to employ hospice staff members who "can accept direction and authority." One said: "People are political and we might as well be realistic about the fact that there is going to be jockeying for power and money as the hospice staff members fight to establish their turf." Since teamwork is at the heart of the hospice concept, those planning a hospice program should therefore make sure that board members, administrators, and all staff persons are publicly committed to the notion that no one person has all the answers, and that the total care of terminally-ill persons requires personnel who can work together and co-operate as equals and partners, and who are resolved to break down inter-professional rivalries and concomitant defensive attitudes in order to create something new.

People whose emotional resources are continually drained through contact with grief and dying, without being adequately replenished, will not long be able to take proper care of dying persons or to sustain the burdens of staff teamwork. Support, however, is more than emotional support from team members and psychiatrist. It also involves the understanding and awareness of the community, especially of those who contribute time, money, and interest. The most important members of that community are other health-care professionals. While a pat on the back is good for morale, more than good intentions is needed. Those planning a hospice organization must have built-in support, not merely financial, for teamwork, so that, in principle at least, everyone involved with the hospice assumes some responsibility for reinforcing the team concept and helping with the enabling function. At the Palliative Care Unit at Royal Victoria Hospital it is assumed that the social worker on the team will, along with the psychiatrist, play a crucial role in team enabling. Those beginning a new hospice program should make sure that they have access to such behavioral science skills, and can begin by seeking to enable a teamwork philosophy to function in all planning and organizational meetings.

Is There a Model?

It is tempting to hospice planners to look for a model which can be copied or duplicated in another community—a facility in Britain, for example, or a hospice home-care program in America. This temptation must be avoided. It is a mistake to think that there is somewhere a model which can be used in order to avoid painstaking local work. At the same time, however, a demonstration model, such as attempted at New Haven, can stimulate the imagination in specific ways. Thus, with detailed information available, a great deal of time and effort can be saved in getting the process started elsewhere. A great deal can be learned from mistakes and failure, as well as from successful experience. Because model building takes much time and skill, the process at New Haven is only just beginning even after some years. And later, what will be found at New Haven Hospice will be a functional model rather than an ideal one. One of the values of a demonstration model lies in the experience of model building itself. Not only do alternative models stimulate the imagination by proposing and clarifying new possibilities and alternatives, but the process of model building itself can be an artistic means for stimulating learning and imaginative evaluation processes. The human failure evidenced in the way many terminally-ill persons are treated in American culture results from one type of failure in human imagination. The hospice models discussed here provide essentially a framework for expanding and enlarging the imagination, the vision of methods, goals, and means for change, for asking basic questions and comparing present possibilities for some directions in which to seek answers.

The hospice that seeks to be a demonstration model, therefore, is not audaciously proposing itself as ideal or even as something to be copied in another community. Instead, it presents itself as an institutional program which seeks to be a research and learning experience not only for itself but also for others across the country. In other words, a model may be designed to clarify issues and to provide a basis for experimentation, with present models being comparable to Model T Fords in the process of demonstrating what the ideal automobile might someday be. For example, many people see no alternatives to the physician-dominated authoritarian styles of health-care institutions simply because they have not had the chance to see and become involved in creative alternatives. It may be interesting and helpful to diagram informal and formal organizational structures, but good administration in a hospice program will primarily be concerned with persons and their growth. If a hospice program is to serve patients and families in more humane and compassionate ways, then from the beginning it should demonstrate in all its procedures a concern for the helpless and ill-informed which will never sacrifice people to goals or expertise. Model building and hospice creating will of necessity have to be realistic about the way things are accomplished in our society. Power exists and must be used to make decisions, to obtain money, to create serving programs. People who have power must therefore be involved in decisions, just as terminally-ill people and their families must be involved in the decisions that affect their care and treatment. Models may be descriptive or predictive—*i.e.*, demonstrating how things are or how they might be. The question is not whether to use models in demonstrations, but how to learn from and how to use the process of model building consistently with the hospice point of view and the sort of program that is needed. That is, no experience or experimentation is above criticism, and significant lessons can be learned from any valid experimentation that takes itself seriously as a model in those terms.

It has been suggested that New Haven Hospice, and perhaps all such programs, should be developed with planned obsolescence as an ultimate goal. Even those who plan to construct hospice facilities should hope that these will not be needed after thirty years. For the "model" idea intends to demonstrate not only better ways of taking care of terminally-ill persons but also to point out one way in which the health-care structures of the country can be helped to move in new directions which will make such hospice services unnecessary, for they will then be implicit in all health-care programs and services.

Consultative Services

During this period while the libraries and resources of existing hospices are limited, and services and counsel to persons in other communities are subject to the availability of staff time, New Haven Hospice sees itself as a resource center for those people who are considering hospices elsewhere. Speakers and consultants are available on a fee basis. From time to time consultations are planned to draw together persons who need to study various aspects of the hospice idea. New Haven Hospice plans to expand its Library Resource Center into a national information service once its new hospice facility is constructed in Branford. At Branford there will be space for study, training, consultation, and observation. It will also be helpful as a place for goal setting, and for research to test different methods of accomplishing goals.

What Can One Person Do?

Initial efforts to stir up community interest with view to getting the hospice idea discussed might come from a physician, nurse or pastor. There are many things that one person can do. Such an initiator might begin by gathering printed material, perhaps even by visiting a hospice program to secure information for use in making talks around the community. A next step would be to call together a group of persons who could begin to study and work together, perhaps following a planning style such as is suggested by DeBoer who defines non-planning style for making decisions as "unanticipated, unpredictable bolts of lightning," in contrast to good planning which stimulates a flow like "electricity through wires and controlled by a switch." [3] Unfortunately, he says, many worthwhile efforts at community initiative fail or else limp along with meager success because the energy of the volunteers is used in ways more similar to the bolts of lightning than to the regularly generated currents of power flowing through the wire.

Planning, even when one is the first and perhaps only one in the community with the idea, should proceed in a systematic rather than in a haphazard way. One should reflect upon how best to get facts, determine goals and objectives, identify alternatives, detail an action plan, set up productive meetings to involve the right people, do long-range planning, and foresee how decisions can be made.[4] The vision is there to be seen, and implementing materials and suggestions are available through any library. As the medical director of the Palliative Care Unit at Royal Victoria Hospital said: "It is a rare privilege to take part in the first tottering steps of an infant discipline."

FOR FURTHER READING

On teamwork: Drummon, H. D., "Team Teaching, An Assessment," *Educational Leadership*, December 1965, Vol. 19; Horowitz, J. J. *Team Practice and the Specialist*. Springfield, Ill.: Charles C Thomas, 1970; Newcomb, Dorothy. *The Team Plan—A Manual for Nursing Services Administration*. New York: G. P. Putnam's Sons, 1971; Swansburg, R. C. *Team Nursing—A Programmed Learning Experience*. New York: G. P. Putnam's Sons, 1968; Rossman, P., "Education in and for Team Ministry," *Christian Century*, Feb. 2, 1970; and "Special Teams Number," *Newsletter*, World Council of Churches, no. 3, March 1969.

9

Some Financial Aspects

Hospice programs, whether home care or in-facility, must be financed for the most part through daily fees paid by patients and their families—that is, in most cases, from private or tax-funded health insurance reimbursement. It is helpful, therefore, to begin by looking at the problem of lingering terminal illness when faced by families like Mrs. Morgan's. When the Social Security program was initiated, it was commonly expected that elderly persons who needed care would be taken into nursing homes for monthly payments close to what the patient would receive from his or her Social Security payments. In the 1960's the American people still had faith that our free-enterprise health-care system was basically sound but that it had just overlooked the poor and the elderly. Several improvements were designed to improve the system; among them Medicare, Medicaid, and neighborhood health centers for the poor.[1] Mrs. Morgan had Social Security and Medicare, so what was her situation?

Mrs. Morgan owned her home, had $20,000 worth of stocks which she and her husband had saved to help finance their grandchildren's college education. She received Social Security payments and that plus her other income totaled about $4,800 a year. One reason she wept in the hospital was that her bills might reach $50,000 a year—more if she required special nursing. Her family had not worried about such costs for Mrs. Morgan because of the common American faith that insurance will cover all. Americans have not taken much thought of what the taxpayer is being charged. But after the first sixty days—which were covered by insurance—Mrs. Morgan's hospital bills took a first leap to $780 a month, or nearly twice her income. Her home had already been mortaged to pay nursing-home bills, so the family was stunned a number of months later to be confronted with bills of over $1,500 a month as their share even before Medicare ran out. (When a member of the family bristled at these charges, the hospital clerk smiled helpfully and said: "You must remember that America offers the best medical care in the world." Whereupon the reply was: "Perhaps Rolls Royce makes the world's best cars, but if there were no other choice, how many of us would ride?")

It was perhaps only right that Mrs. Morgan's house was sold, along with all of her furniture and possessions, in order to pay these bills. Although it must be said that to have this done before she died was a source of great anguish to Mrs. Morgan. As do most people, she had certain souvenirs and pieces of furniture that she wanted to keep, and she suffered at the thought of how they were being handled. But the unfair financial burden fell harder upon Mrs. Morgan's daughter Emma, who quit her job and gave up her rented home in another city in order to look after her mother. Emma worked for over two years without salary in taking care of her mother and it was exhausting work. By rights Emma should have inherited her mother's house in exchange for this care so that she would have had a place to live when she herself was old. Instead, she went to work clerking in a store when her mother went into the hospital and spent every penny she could spare on her mother's care. Emma, as a result of helping with her share of Mrs. Morgan's hospital costs, was rapidly aging and with no savings of her own. There seemed to be no way for Mrs. Morgan to be cared for in hospital, nursing home, or in her own home, without Emma's being financially crushed—she had no life or future of her own. Mrs. Morgan's health insurance did not provide adequately for home care, even though to have kept her at home would have saved large sums in tax revenues.

Why Higher Costs?

It would be a mistake to think that Mrs. Morgan's high hospital costs were the result of the medical profession's seeking to enrich itself at her expense. Her own physician, in fact, submitted only very modest bills and always told Mrs. Morgan's daughter to take as long as she needed to pay them. Nor did any of the specialists who were incolved in Mrs. Morgan's cancer care ever raise any question of payment, even though their costs were for the most part covered by insurance. Still, in the over-all picture, medical expenses such as drugs, physicians' fees, and hospital bills increased ten times between 1950 and 1974,[2] with the result that the American middle class was almost priced out of the health-care marketplace when they found themselves with lingering illnesses like Mrs. Morgan's. Why? The University of Pennsylvania Health Law Project found that—as always seems inevitable with government programs—the amount of paperwork multiplied to take up nearly 70 per cent of the funds set aside for persons like Mrs. Morgan. As a result of forms to be filled out, keeping files, making reports, and financing the bureaucracy, Medicaid costs increased three times faster than the number of persons served between 1968 and 1970, for example. Health care became more expensive, more complicated, and its costs escalated even more than American military costs, with "no precedent for any similar sustained expansion in any other sector of the civilian economy." [3]

The costs multiplied because the American people had decided to declare war on disease, and when a society is at war it gives less attention to scrutinizing the budget requests of its leaders in the struggle. Also, as in any war there always are people who use the war to serve their own interests. Some physicians and drug producers became privateers, enriching themselves as a result of the war on disease. But even this was for the most part the result of the full-speed-ahead, win-the-war-at-any-cost attitude. When a country is under attack the army gets what it asks for. Thus the availability of tax funds and of prepaid insurance, with the attendant public enthusiasm, encouraged health-care administrators into self-indulgence and led to the provision of far more medical technology than many communities needed, and often too many hospital beds as well. Schwartz, for example, asks if every hospital needs, and if every community should be asked to pay for, computerized axial tomography.[4] This computerized equipment for diagnosis can cost from $250,000 to $600,000, with the cost prorated to hospital bills of patients like Mrs. Morgan who never need or use the equipment. Schwartz warns that unless brakes are applied, American hospitals—often duplicating equipment already available in another hospital in town—will purchase 10 to 18 billion dollars' worth of such technology, charging it off to patients and taxpayers who were never adequately consulted and who probably will make little use of it.

Mushrooming paper work and vast expenditures for technology have served to escalate costs for patients like Mrs. Morgan, in part because of the very insurance plans which were designed to take the burden of such costs from her. The availability of government programs seems to mitigate against economy and careful planning in many cases. Geiger notes further that Federal and state insurance programs are administered by Blue Cross, a private agency which in turn is controlled by the hospitals themselves.[5] In other words, "What happens when the fox is not merely in the chicken coop, but is appointed by the government to be its administrator?" Institutions or foxes, he says, are not necessarily evil, but they will tend first to look after their own interests and survival. He points to the well-documented fact that the "reasonable cost formula" for determining hospital charges "has nothing to do with what is reasonable by any market or accounting standard." Hospitals, he says, can charge off to Medicare not only drugs, supplies and medical equipment which may be purchased at higher-than-necessary prices, but they can also charge to Medicare a portion of their public relation costs designed to present a good public image. In other words, the interests even of benevolent institutions like hospitals do not necessarily coincide with the public interest. Human beings tend to run institutions to serve their own interests unless accountability is built into the system. Geiger therefore proposes that consumers must be elected to the boards of directors of Blue Cross, as well as to more hospital boards. Otherwise, he says, a national comprehensive insurance program, when Congress passes one, will be a "great leap sideways" that will continue to provide insurance for hospitals, *not patients.*

The hospice concept seeks to help patients control their own lives and the institutions and programs upon which they depend. At the moment this can perhaps best be accomplished by keeping more patients, especially the terminally ill, out of impersonal institutions as much as possible. Certainly, if hospital costs are to be kept high in order to marshal technology in a war on disease, then people who can no longer be cured should be moved out of that system and kept out. American society may soon find itself in the precarious situation of spending millions of dollars per person to keep large numbers of patients alive on machines for many years even though they never will be conscious again. If it costs $50,000 to $75,000 a year to take care of a conscious and alert patient like Mrs. Morgan, how much more will it cost to keep hundreds of thousands of persons on machines? At some point the society of the future must make fundamental decisions about when to let people die or otherwise all the resources of society could go into keeping unconscious people alive. Hospitals already face such decisions to a limited extent, as they decide upon vast sums for technology for the few, to be charged against the bills of the many.

Lower Costs at Home

In any case, no matter how much hospital costs are controlled, it is obvious that society could save a great deal of money by taking care of many patients at home. The New Haven Hospice, when it erects its new facility, hopes to demonstrate lower per diem facility costs, because a hospice facility need not purchase and maintain the expensive technical equipment that adds so much to the cost of a hospital bed. St. Christopher's Hospice has found it useful to have a resuscitator—but for the occasional use of visitors, not patients. A hospice facility needs only to have simple equipment and a homelike atmosphere. With patients and their families as partners in their own care, costs can be further reduced. It has therefore been estimated that even if costs in a hospice facility were as high as $102 a day—as compared to $200 a day at a New Haven hospital—the nation's insurance bill for terminally-ill patients could be reduced by one third to one half, with a resultant saving of billions of dollars.

Also there are other savings to be achieved. An expert on bereavement has demonstrated that significant savings on costs for psychiatric care and mental hospitals for survivors can be achieved by preventive counseling with the bereaved, an important aspect of the total hospice program.[6] The cost of untreated bereavement to the community also includes drugs like tranquilizers, as well as alcohol use. It has been found that proper bereavement counseling at the right moment can reduce other medical costs among survivors. Some bereavement care within the context of a hospice team can often be accomplished by unpaid hospice volunteers, whereas later it would involve expensive psychiatric costs.

It is in the area of home care, however, that New Haven Hospice is able to demonstrate the most dramatic financial saving for society and for families. In some situations Medicare is now able to pay only 40 per cent of the medical bills, and this percentage has been decreasing. Mrs. Morgan's large hospital bills could have been reduced to a point where her pension would have paid a large share of costs if she had been kept at home. And the burden to her insurance would have been much more manageable to society if home care—including physician, nursing assistance, counseling and all the services of a hospice team—could be provided for half of what it would cost to keep her in a medical facility. Thus making a saving for society of billions of dollars. And, most ironically, the care that Mrs. Morgan could have afforded would have made her a million times happier! Based upon an analysis of sources of reimbursement for 923 patients who died at Yale-New Haven Hospital, one estimate suggests that a New Haven Hospice facility could be available to all persons who need its services with reimbursement approximately as follows:

Medicare	45–50%
Blue Cross	27%
Medicaid	10–12%
Private Insurance	12%
Other sources (military, child health, special grants)	2%

Since the average length of stay of a terminally-ill patient in a hospital was found to be twenty-one days, hospitalization costs in 1973 averaged between $2,187 and $3,385 on a rate per day of $104 to $161. Had a hospice facility been operating in New Haven in 1973, its daily rate could have been $84 or less. A twenty-one day stay in the hospice would therefore have resulted in clearly demonstrable *cost savings* of between $424 and $1,622 per patient, without accounting for further reduction in cost for any periods of time the patient was aided by the hospice to stay at home. And, for someone like Mrs. Morgan who lived much longer in her terminal period, the savings would have escalated tremendously.

As Garner has pointed out,[7] the debate on relative costs is going to require more research and experience before it is complete. The Palliative Care Unit at Royal Victoria Hospital has been able to demonstrate to Quebec Government officials that the hospice program saved the hospital nearly $200,000 in 1975. Patients dying from cancer at Royal Victoria Hospital spent an average of thirty-three days as in-patients before dying, frequently occupying the high-cost intensive care space at the hospital. The home-care program of the Palliative Care Unit reduced the cost per family and increased the number of persons that could be served by one bed in the Unit by 35 per month in 1969–70, and by 49 per month in 1973. The savings to the hospital were in fact more than that, as long as hospital beds also remained full of other patients. An analysis of home-care cases for a three-month period (April–June, 1976) showed that the average patient was saving $80 a day, and the hospital was saving $130,900 for the period, even when home-care costs were estimated to be as high as $100 a day.[8] The research report pointed out that 75 to 80 per cent of hospital expense consists of salaries, and savings in a palliative care program depend on salary costs. Nursing costs were higher for patients in the hospice program, averaging out to $9.65 more per day per patient for those hospitalized; but savings in laboratory costs and costs of services that were routine in other sections of the hospital more than compensated for these costs, suggesting that a hospice program can save money even when it is contained within a general hospital. The home-care program, though not intended as a money-saving device, is nevertheless also cheaper, as also demonstrated in Great Britain at St. Christopher's Hospice, where the stay of a patient is from 15 days to three months.

On the basis of experimentation and its unit of cost study, the New Haven Hospice as of the fall of 1978 had determined a fee of $29 per home visit. The Hospice's first effort was to recover as much of this amount as possible from Medicare which Hospice is able to do as a Certified Home Health Agency, from Medicaid (Title XIX), from Blue Cross of Connecticut, with which Hospice has a good contract, and from the private insurance companies. Hospice also has a Title XX grant providing services to people of lower income, and a Title III grant which makes it possible to provide services to older citizens. If a patient is not covered by any of these programs, a sliding scale is then applied. No one is ever turned away for lack of money. In other communities a Visiting Nurse Association may charge from $16 to $50 a visit depending on many factors—including whether or not it is adequately subsidized to help poor families, the extent of staff services it can provide, and so on. Some associations employ nurses who are clinical specialists; others use licensed practical nurses. Some associations offer physical therapy along with other services. New Haven Hospice has been able to offer its home-care program at no cost to the family during a pilot experimental period funded by the National Cancer Institute, which is thus making possible a thorough study to help determine what home care is going to cost and the savings it can provide for the community.

From March 1974 until October 1, 1978, the New Haven Hospice Home Care Program had served 585 patients and families with full scope services. (463 had died, 279 or 59 per cent at home.) During the 1977-78 fiscal year 74 per cent died at home. The daily caseload consisted of approximately 35 patient/families and 35 bereaved families. For the most part the 110 physicians who had made referrals to the hospice program were oncologists. Data for cost planning will be available from the New Haven Hospice's retrieval system, which consists of the Hospice Home Care Patient/Family Profile, the Hospice Home Care Service Profile, the Staff Time Allocation Record, and the Telephone Usage Record. The system is designed to answer basic questions such as how the Hospice Home Care Program has met its specific objectives, and how Hospice Home Care patient and family population differs from non-Hospice patient care and family population. Such information is not at present available from any other source.[9]

In-facility Reimbursement

As hearings proceeded during initial stages of program development, the Connecticut health planning staff assured the directors of New Haven Hospice that Federal government programs like Medicare would, "subject to Federal regulations," reimburse the hospice once its facility was constructed and licensed as a chronic disease hospital. It quickly became clear, however, that certain aspects of the total hospice program—such as bereavement counseling—are not at present provided for under such regulations. Connecticut state law provides for the licensing and inspecting of all clinics, hospitals, and skilled nursing facilities; for the regulation of hospital rates and construction; and for receiving and administering Federal Title XIX funds. What is done by state officials is therefore complicated by Federal regulations. In this context New Haven Hospice had to decide how to apply for recognition as an entity within state and Federal law—a difficult situation since it was not a general hospital, nor a psychiatric hospital, nor a chronic disease facility, and did not fit into the types of institutions thus defined as qualified for reimbursement. The hospice board of directors gave thought to encouraging political action to get state laws revised, but had to be realistic in the immediate adjustment to possibilities. The hospice concept posed a number of difficult problems in relation to legal regulations. For example, reimbursers did not want to hear anything at all about "care for *patient-and-family*," a concept so basic to the hospice program. Unless each member of the family was individually covered by Medicare, Medicaid, or some insurance program, services could not be provided for all members of the family.

The type of license a hospice facility applied for would also greatly determine the rate of reimbursement, setting a precedent for other such hospice programs. The $15 to $25 a day which most states allow for nursing homes is not adequate to maintain a hospice-type facility; yet how could the hospice qualify for hospital rates? A new standard was needed between nursing homes and hospitals to be used for specialized terminal-care facilities. Perhaps 50 per cent of hospice costs were reimbursable under present regulations once the legal knots were patiently untied through negotiation, for the savings that a hospice facility represents speak a language of economies which politicians and bureaucrats can hear and understand. Hospice applied to the Connecticut Department of Health for a special category entitled "Short-term Hospital—Special: Hospice."

Home-Care Reimbursement

Reimbursement of home-care services faced similar obstacles, although as of August 21, 1975, there were changes in the Federal law which made it mandatory for each state to offer skilled home-care nursing and equipment (Regulation 45-C-FR-5249). It is significant that at a time when the Federal government was cutting back on nearly all programs it was wanting to expand home care. In some states, such as New York, New Mexico, and Connecticut, the law also made it mandatory for private group health insurance plans to provide financial assistance for home care, suggesting that first steps were under way to clear the way for reimbursement for hospice-type programs. However, even where insurance plans are providing some home-care reimbursement, the feature is rarely advertised or pointed out to purchasers. This may be due in part to the fact that the insurance companies are not yet quite sure as to what may be involved in home-care services, and since the motivation for home care comes from the fact that it is cheaper, abuses in the program may occur as in hospitals. A staff member from the Connecticut Department of Health recently told a hospice consultation that in actual practice Federal regulations make it possible for a specific state to do only very little even if it wishes to do more, and suggested that citizen political action will be necessary in many states to secure better provision for programs for the terminally ill.

In any case, reimbursement does not provide for dental care, for bereavement care, or for many of the social work functions of a hospice home-care program. Hospices therefore face specific problems in understanding where to move within the framework of existing law. For example, can a licensed practical nurse give certain medication and tests? If a hospice applied for licensing as an independent home-care health agency under Medicaid and Medicare, it would be necessary to cut back the program to fit into regulations which are at present too limited and inadequate for comprehensive terminal care. If a hospice were so licensed it could qualify for funds and could also receive a recognized place within the structure for certifying supervisory personnel, for defining limits of program and services. It would be easy for a hospice to say: "We are innovating and need not worry yet about how we can qualify under government regulations until we get well established," without realizing that preliminary steps may lock up the future of the program. The present time, when many states are making changes in reimbursement policy, provides a crucial opportunity for hospices to influence these changes.

The 1978 Connecticut Legislature changed policies which had discriminated against the terminally ill, changing the law which had mandated reimbursement for home care only "(1) if continued hospitalization would otherwise have been required if home care was not provided, and (2) the plan covering home care is established and approved in writing by such physician within seven days following termination of hospital confinement as a resident in-patient for the same or related condition for which the covered person was hospitalized, and (3) such home care is commenced within seven days following discharge."[10] In other words, a patient could not move in and out of a hospice and have home care covered during intervening periods, and home care is designed to taper off as a person discharged from a hospital gets well. The 1975 law provided for no bereavement care, social work assistance (which is provided in 1978), or family care and would pay for more than one month of care only under conditions which did not apply to the terminally ill. As hospice staff have found over and over again, the real problem may well be the nonrecognition of the problem on the part of persons who should be informed, and, as a result, most people who die today are already ruled out by existing law, defined out by institutional policy. Is this going to improve or get worse as the percentage of aged in the population increases? Conwell, for example, worries that by 1990 the number of black women in the over-85 age category will increase by 215 per cent, and that the use of pure cost-benefit analysis will probably cause society to alter the allocation of public funds to favor the young over the old, the educated over the uneducated, the rich over the poor, and to downgrade concern over chronic illness, unless the direction is changed now before it is too late.[11] In this situation more and more people are feeling that better care for less can be provided for more people at home, but for the terminally ill this means additional changes in the law.

Constructing a Facility

However in-facility programs and home care may be financed, New Haven Hospice faced a large-scale fund-raising program before a facility could be constructed. As of November 1978, $412,892 had been raised, with $294,044 from individuals,

$50,348 from corporations, and $68,500 from foundations. With the land purchased, the cost for construction will be $3,500,000, and the hospice board of directors explored alternative plans for proceeding. One possibility was funding from the Public Works Employment Act of 1976, which would require deeding the property to the town of Branford, which would in turn apply to the Federal government for funds. Under this plan the town would lease the building to the hospice for ninety-nine years. A second possibility was to issue bonds through a corporate trust to be managed by a New Haven bank. The bonds would be floated for a 25-year term at the rate of 5 per cent per annum, and the issue would be offered to religious organizations which have investment portfolios. This plan was being explored and developed by banking consultants who have volunteered their time to the hospice. A third alternative was to float bonds through the Connecticut Hospital and Educational Facilities Authority, with bonds in either case amounting to $2,250,000. Other communities, as they investigate various plans for hospice facilities, can profit from these imaginative possibilities and will no doubt find other innovative ways of raising funds.

A federal grant of $1,000,000 and a state grant of $1,500,000 made possible an autumn, 1977, ground breaking for the Hospice in New Haven county.

It is clear, however, that the basic hospice program objective of lowering the cost for the care of the terminally ill will not be achieved in any adequate way except as enabling legislation is passed in state capitals and until national health insurance plans are defined and acted upon in Washington. Meanwhile, the most satisfactory arrangement for an increasing number of terminal patients will be to remain at home with the burden of expense shared by health insurance plans.

FOR FURTHER READING: See also: R. W. Hetherington et al. Health Insurance Plans: Performance and Promise (New York: Wiley, 1975); Richard Lyons, "The Challenges to the Doctors," New York Times, June 29, 1974; "Liberal Benefits," in Geriatrics, January 1976.

Home Care for the Dying

Home care for the elderly, the sick, and the handicapped—in preference to institutional care—is a concept which is going to be explored thoroughly in the next decade. The issue is more complicated, however, than may appear at first glance. It involves controversial matters with unions, plus proposals that family members be employed to care for relatives. From the perspective of patient and family, the issue involves deeper meanings than adequate physical care. Therefore this chapter, addressed primarily to family members, must consist of far more than advice and a recital of techniques. Home care is an aspect of a major new movement in medicine which aims to keep patients in control of their own lives as much as possible, just as good health care requires individuals to assume responsibility for their own health.

Some families are accustomed to living on welfare and accepting all kinds of help from charitable agencies and organizations. Other families, typical of many in the middle class, may not even be aware of the range of social services available to them in a crisis. Surprisingly, they often feel that it is like "accepting charity" to ask for guidance and help. If Mrs. Morgan's family, for example, had been better informed of services available to them, they could have been far more self-reliant in taking care of Mrs. Morgan at home as she wished. The ongoing shift of more responsibility to the family and patient is illustrated dramatically in the new procedures for dialysis in kidney disease. Whereas at one time all such patients were closely dependent on kidney machines at hospitals, a new portable unit which the patient can use at home is saving the taxpayers hundreds of millions of dollars that would otherwise be required to multiply dialysis centers. At the same time, and more important, it is giving the kidney patient a new freedom, and a renewed self-responsibility along with his or her family.[1] By the same token, the hospice program enters into the life of a terminally-ill patient/family to offer a similar independence.

The Home Care Program of New Haven Hospice begins as a relationship to the family which is established with the first telephone call of inquiry when some member of the family reaches out to ask for help. The first response by the hospice staff member who answers the phone is personal and expresses concern. Every effort is then made either to keep the patient at home as long as possible or to take the patient home from the hospital as the case may be. The needs of any specific patient may require some time to be spent in a hospital or nursing home, but the basic need is not to minimize medical care but to maximize it—to bring all the best of medical knowledge to bear upon patients so they can return home to live out their remaining weeks in comfort. The home-care team brings a variety of services to bear in assisting the family to make this possible.

Hospice Home-Care Services

The extent and kind of service the hospice will provide depends upon level of need—from full service to medical consultation on pain control, from nursing consultation on the management of a patient at home to counseling relatives. Full service in the home setting consists essentially of visits and attention from a physician for palliative care, regular nursing visits (with additional visits on call as needed, 24-hours a day and 7-days-a week). Private duty nursing is not provided, and weekday physical care is often arranged in collaboration with the local Visiting Nurse Association or Public Health Nursing Association. A third component of home care is social work consultation with families and patient. A fourth is pastoral-care consultation direct or arranged through the patient's pastor, priest, or rabbi. Volunteers are available as friendly visitors, to assist with shopping, sitting, with transportation, and so on. And, finally, bereavement care is provided.

Every Tuesday the entire home-care staff of New Haven Hospice meets to discuss each patient and family thoroughly, to refine the plan of care in each case, and to make sure that no needs are overlooked. Each patient is assigned a primary nurse, and regular nursing visits are made to assist and counsel the family. Consultation is provided primarily by the social worker, nurse, or physician discussing and evaluating the practical problems which the family faces. Members of the family often come to the hospice office for such advice. Hospice nurses provide instruction and advice on the care of a terminally-ill patient; and these services are made available within a ten-town geographical area. For example, a family may need help in dealing with pain or discomfort, or in the middle of the night may need advice on nursing procedures. Members of the hospice team can also provide advice and counsel on diet, food preparation and feeding of a patient; suggestions for recreation and diversion for the patient if the home has limited resources; and they can help find needed equipment, whether it be a hospital bed, wheelchair, or whatever. As the family and patient come to know and trust the hospice team, many other questions, important and unimportant, will emerge which the team will help to answer.

Patient Advocacy

Even families who know that physicians usually call in consultants and consider alternatives in difficult medical cases, often uncritically accept the first medical advice which is given to them. Many families fail to inform themselves of alternative medical care which may be available. A good many families of cancer patients, for example, are finding that a patient gets better treatment if patient and family carefully inform themselves of what is to be done and carefully watch the process step by step. In reviewing *Julia's Story*,[2] a book about a woman who died of neglect after surgery, Jean Brodie says that while it is not the sort of book one would want to read before entering the hospital for an operation,[3] it is a useful example of medical neglect and of family failure to challenge health-care personnel—a story which can be duplicated over and over again. In *Julia's Story* the author tells how his wife had open-heart surgery to replace a damaged valve. The operation was highly successful, but she died after surgery because someone failed to give her the right blood-thinning medicine. The operation was a success, but the patient died. In this case the patient told physicians and nurses that she had "bubbles in her head," which described symptoms that should have alerted them to the problem in time to give her the needed medication. But no one prevented her death because all were busy, care was fragmented, specialists treated part of the patient without being adequately concerned with the whole human being, and most important: 1) there was a lack of teamwork and inadequate consultation between the health-care professionals who were caring for the woman operated upon, and 2) *no one adequately informed the family* of potential dangers so they could be alert for symptoms or problems to call to the attention of nurses and physicians.

Since there are such gaps and loopholes in the present health-care system to which families must be alert, one medical-school professor has, in confidence, suggested that families may in many cases need an advocate to represent them in asking hard questions and enforcing their right to be fully informed of treatment decisions and procedures. The hospice concept provides for such advocacy by including the family, the clergyman, and others as members of the caring team.

Pain Control at Home

In terminal cases it is often in the area of pain control that a family most needs such advocacy and more information. The sections on pain control in this book are not intended fully to inform any family or lay person about proper pain-care procedures, but they do include sufficient detail to make it possible for family members to have a better understanding of what is possible: that terminally-ill persons can in most cases be kept completely free of pain; and that if such is not the case the family should persist in its questions and search for advocacy. In most cases, patients and families will not remember the names of drugs and medicines, much less their nature and functions, but they can certainly grasp the fact that different combinations of medication can be experimented with to meet the varied and complicated needs of a specific patient, in contrast to the practice of many physicians who simply prescribe a tablet of codeine or similar drug every four hours, or use some other equally inflexible form of pain treatment. If the family prepares itself and informs itself diligently for intelligent co-operation with physicians and nurses, most dying persons can be helped to spend comfortable, alert, happy lives for their last days, with self-respect, self-control, freedom, independence and dignity instead of a limiting preoccupation with suffering that drives all meaning from life.

At the same time families need to understand that drugs alone are not enough. Pain control includes back rubs, occupational therapy, talking books, radio and TV, and someone to talk with, since "diversional activity does more than just 'pass the time,' it also diminishes the pain." [4] Twycross points out that the Nazis well understood that torture was most acute and effective when it was meaningless and apparently purposeless. A patient who perceives a universe as senseless and so painful as to demand his total attention finds it much more difficult to cope with pain and stress. [4]

Much pain may be psychological, related to a fear of dying, which Duncombe finds to be best removed by discovering the meaning of one's life, and a coping with a sense of incompleteness about things. [5] At the end of life many persons psychologically need the chance to bring their lives to fruition, to accomplish at least in their reflections about life some measure of fulfillment. "My dream for a hospice," Duncombe says, "is to see it become the place, the occasion, where these deeper life purposes are discovered." In any case, pain is diminished for many persons at the end of life as they are helped to sum up their lives, and overcome their fears and problems. Duncombe feels that many new possibilities are open to the terminally ill because of the new possibilities of pain cure.

At the same time, understanding drugs need not be so complicated as its terminology and ordinary medical procedures suggest. Family members who wish to be well informed so as to monitor and participate in care, can in fact understand as much as they need to know in most situations. For example, how to be alert for signs of pain, and when to summon a nurse or doctor to deal with pain problems.

Nursing Procedures

Other aspects of nursing can be mastered at home, also, and can be accomplished with the guidance of visiting nurses. In addition to dealing with pain, good nursing care involves dealing with nausea, gas, constipation, diarrhea, and other symptoms. For example, a hospice nurse can assist the family in dealing with frequently-neglected mouth problems: ill-fitting dentures or a cracked mouth which may accompany medication. Calvary Hospital in the Bronx developed a mouth-care procedure for coating the tongue and dry areas with a bit of mineral oil and milk of magnesia, a procedure which in a very short time can help patients to enjoy eating and drinking again. Or dry-mouth discomfort can be alleviated, as at St. Luke's, with lemon and glycerin swabs plus ice chips if the patient is conscious.

But while there are many such simple palliative treatments which a family can learn, much nursing attention is expended in simply talking to the patient, touching a hand, expressing affection in other ways, brushing the hair, and so on. Families can, of course, easily be instructed in taking temperature, pulse rate, blood pressure, monitoring lung functioning, and even dialysis, but the first priorities and most common needs are those aspects of simple body care—sanitizing, emptying a bed pan, bathing, changing beds, moving a patient—which can be even more easily learned. Whether terminally-ill patients are old or young, their care includes music, games, and whatever else is possible to enrich a patient's final weeks of life. In one case, it was reported that a patient who knew her time was limited had gained some time through chemotherapy. She was ready to go home but the failure of her family to handle the matter psychologically left her in bed, discouraged and listless. When the family was helped to have a different attitude, however, through hospice counseling, the patient again responded to the clarity and candor of the persons caring for her, rallying round to have some happy weeks. When one speaks of the importance of environment for the terminally ill, therefore, one is perhaps more than anything else expressing a concern for the attitudes and behavior of other members of the family who regularly see and help care for the patient.

Principles of Care

New Haven Hospice has adopted the following principles of care for the terminally-ill patient and family.

- The patient needs to be as symptom-free as possible so that energy can be used to live. The goal of skilled health care is optimum relief of noxious symptoms so that the patient and family can be alert, comfortable, and themselves.
- Terminal illness upsets the equilibrium of the family group. Help is available to all involved, whether patient, relative, or friend.
- The patient/family life-style is disrupted by multiple change. Continuity of care shall be sustained by the same health-care team regardless of locale.
- The patient/family thrives best when its own life-style is maintained and life philosophies respected. The structure of the care system must provide multiple options available to the patient/family under the care of the same health team in different settings.
- Loneliness and isolation are significant sources of anguish to patients who are dying. Care-givers must always be available *where* and *when* the patient needs them.
- The varied problems and anxieties associated with terminal illness can occur at any time, day or night. Therefore 24-hour-a-day care must be available for the patient/family whatever the problem may be.
- The patient/family are needed in making decisions. Education and counseling of the staff and patient/family are required to facilitate communication, share knowledge, and reach decisions.
- No one person can fully meet all the needs of the terminally-ill patient. Care requires collaboration of many disciplines and persons, working as a health-care team.
- The problems of the patient/family facing terminal illness include a wide variety of issues—psychologic, legal, social, spiritual, economic, and interpersonal. Teams must be custom-made and call upon persons and institutions in the community in addition to patient/family and hospice staff.
- Caring for the patient/family as human beings affects

the psychologic state. The staff shall integrate humanistic care with expert medical and nursing care.

- Those who face separation and the end of life need spiritual support. The religious, philosophic, and humanistic components of care are as essential as the medical, nursing, and social work components.

- The patient/family facing death needs someone who cares, and this requires emotional investment on the part of the staff. Such involvement by the staff must be fostered, and the staff given support so that it can sustain involvement.

- Caring involves receiving as well as giving. The patient/family and staff will be educated to act within this principle.

- Emotional investment will cause staff to grieve at the time of loss. Replenishment must be provided through mutual support.

- The environment affects the individual's course in health and disease. The milieu will be designed to make the patient/family condition optimal.[6]

Hospice as Prophetic

Families can share not only in the care of the terminally ill but also in the extension of the hospice concept as a prophetic idea—prophetic in the sense of critical, supportive judgment upon those who would treat human beings impersonally. A medieval hospice was a community of people with a common goal: to care for travelers on the way. The term was thus chosen for this new program because the terminally ill are people who need to find rest and refreshment for concluding their journey of life.

It is important to repeat that while hospices may be shifting attitudes in some hospitals, may indeed be working some changes in the entire health-care system, there must also be a shift in the priorities of society itself if human life is to be valued and enriched. It is ironic that we die poorly because we live poorly. Regardless of whatever criticisms one may mount of the health-care system, it must be said that it reflects the nature of western society and its present priorities. There are many predictions of new approaches to health care which will be preventive, and a society where illness will hardly exist, where persons will not be institutionalized, but, instead will be personalized.[7] In this connection, Powledge has said of hospices: "Most people will not die in such a place, but their going may be easier because of things learned there." [8]

How does a lay person become interested in devoting time and money to the development of a hospice? As an example, a nephew stopped recently to visit a favorite uncle who had been many months dying in an urban hospital. The nephew and his wife had crossed the country by car and they had discussed how fortunate their uncle was to live in a city with such excellent medical facilities. Living elsewhere, they agreed, the uncle would already have died.

When they came out of the hospital, however, after their first visit, the nephew and his wife sat in their car shaken and dismayed.

"I'm sorry we came," the wife said. For the uncle, strapped to a bed to prevent him from committing suicide, was attached to a machine and was twitching miserably. He had begged his nephew to help him die. "Is this what he saved his money for?" the wife added.

The nephew shook his head, remembering his uncle's plans for security and happiness in his old age. "What haunts me is the misery in Uncle's eyes. I remember a prison book which described the fiendish tortures of a sadistic guard, who would strap a helpless convict to a bed until the prisoner went mad. Some strong convicts could stand it for weeks, but Uncle has been this way for longer than that."

Disturbed, wondering what to do, the nephew and his wife met by chance a woman whose father had, in a similar situation, become so depressed that he wouldn't talk to anyone.

When it first became possible for a hospice team to assist him, he had not even been willing to talk to the nurse. Gradually, however, the team had been able, through patience and affection, to take him to a garden where he could watch children play. He began to talk to the nurse and then to open up to the staff. He lived longer than expected away from his machine. He began to ask for his favorite foods, and wanted to play cards. He was even able to go home briefly.

The hospice concept is seen in the contrast between those two patients who illustrate the sense in which it is prophetic. Both visionary and practical, it enables an increasing number of persons to die happily, often at home, "protected from the institutional encroachments upon their dignity, maintaining their individuality, staying close to family and loved ones." [9] The hospice program provides the opportunity for family, patient, and community to confront the problem of dying with honesty, "to diminish the suffering associated with dying— both for the patient and for his family—and thereby to ease bereavement." By teaching hospice staff, "patients create something that will live after their death . . . and by sharing their experience of dying . . . patients enable hospice staff members to surmount the denial of death that so often is taught—a denial which enables us to tolerate the inhuman vegetation that is the hallmark of superfluousness among the terminally ill of America," making possible a "humanizing of the process of dying—by consecrating death as a part of life." [10]

FOR FURTHER READING

Stroller, J. H. *Home Care*. Boston: Little, Brown and Co., 1975; McNulty, R. J., "Discharging the Terminally Ill Patient," *Nursing Times*, Sept. 10, 1970; Kerppola-Sirola, I., "The Death of an Old Professor," *Journal of the American Medical Association*, May 1975; Klinger, J. L. *et al. Mealtime Manual for the Aged and*

Hospitalized. New York: Simon and Shuster; Asbury, Edith, "Health Care in Home Supported for Aged, but Only if Closely Monitored," *New York Times*, Sept. 21, 1976.

And recommended: *American Red Cross Home Nursing Textbook*. New York: Doubleday and Company; and *Home Nursing Handbook* from the Metropolitan Life Insurance Co., One Madison Ave., New York, N.Y. 10010. Single copies of the latter are free upon request.

Chapter Notes

Introduction

1. Constance Holden. "Hospices: For the Dying, Relief from Pain and Fear," *Science*, Vol. 193, July 30, 1976, pp. 389 ff.
2. Cicely Saunders. "The Last Frontier," in R. B. Reeves, *et al. Pastoral Care of the Dying and the Bereaved: Selected Readings* (New York: Health Sciences Publishing Corp., 1973).
3. Elisabeth Kübler-Ross. *On Death and Dying* (New York: Macmillan Co., 1969).
4. R. Lamerton. "Care of the Dying—Teamwork," *Nursing Times*, Dec. 28, 1972, Vol. 68, no. 52.
5. Parker Rossman. "A Prophetic Ministry to the Dying," *Christian Century*, Apr. 21, 1976.
6. *Ibid.*
7. *Ibid.*
8. *Newsweek*, Jan. 6, 1975.
9. C. S. Lewis, *A Grief Observed* (New York: Seabury Press, 1961), p. 61.
10. Rossman, *op. cit.*

Chapter 1. Mrs. Morgan Wanted to Die at Home

1. All names are changed and Mrs. Alma Morgan is a composite case which combines elements from three cases in as many different states so that no one can be embarrassed by recognition.
2. Elisabeth Kübler-Ross. *On Death And Dying* (New York: Macmillan Co., 1969), paperback. See also from the same publisher her *Questions and Answers About Death and Dying* (1971), and *Death: The Final Stage of Growth* (1975).
3. See, for example: Chapter IV on the right to refuse treatment,

in R. M. Veatch, *Death, Dying, and the Biological Revolution* (New Haven: Yale University Press, 1976); George Annas, *et al.*, "The Patient's Rights Advocate," *Vanderbilt Law Review*, 1974, pp. 243 ff.; Robert Chiles, "The Rights of Patients," *New England Journal of Medicine*, 1967, pp 411 ff.; Derrone, "Do Patients Have Rights," *Trial*, 1973, pp. 59 ff.

4. Veatch, *op. cit.*

5. See, for example, the "Living Will," recommended by the Euthanasia Educational Fund, 250 West 57th St., New York, N.Y. 10019.

6. In Stanley E. Troup, William A. Green, *et al. The Patient, Death, and the Family* (New York: Charles Scribner's Sons, 1974).

7. In Sylvia Lack and Richard Lamerton. *The Hour of Death—A Record of a Conference on the Care of the Dying* (London: Geoffrey Chapman, 1974).

8. Melvin J. Krant. *Dying and Dignity* (Springfield, Ill.: Charles C Thomas, 1974). pp. 33 ff.

Chapter 2. The Dilemma of the Family

1. Richard Lamerton. *Care of the Dying*. (London: Priority Press, 1973), page 40.

2. Philosopher Huston Smith of M.I.T. discusses such a perspective in Troup and Green, *op. cit.*, p. 19.

3. Private communication to author.

4. "Helping Families to Cope," *Internal Medicine News,* Aug. 1, 1976.

5. "Informing Cancer Patient," *Internal Medicine News*, Aug. 1, 1976.

6. C. M. Parkes. *Bereavement* (New York: International Universities Press, 1972).

7. *Ibid.*

8. Edward F. Dobihal, "Talk of Terminal Care," *Connecticut Medicine*, July 1974, p. 365.

9. *Ibid.*

Chapter 3. Health-Care Professionals and the Dying

1. Krant, *Dying and Dignity*, *op. cit.*, p. 3.

2. See John Knowles, "The Hospital," *Scientific American*, September 1973.

3. From an unpublished study by David Duncombe, chaplain of

Yale Medical School, and Chase Kimball. Yeates Conwell, in an unpublished paper, "Toward an Ideal System of Care for the Terminally Ill," submitted as a Senior Thesis at Princeton, cites evidence from several sources that physicians fear death more than do their patients. Also, A. M. Kasper, "The Doctor and Death," in H. Feifel, ed., *The Meaning of Death* (New York: McGraw Hill, 1959), found that the fear of death was an element in the choice of medicine as a career.

4. Krant, *op. cit.*, p. 45.

5. Barbara M. Stewart, "Living With Cancer," *Nursing Forum*, Vol. 13, no. 1, 1974, p. 53.

6. Conwell, *op. cit.*, p. 77.

7. Krant, *op cit.*, p. 75.

8. D. Mechanic, "Social Psychologic Factors affecting the Presentation of Bodily Complaints," *Politics, Medicine, and Social Science* (New York: John Wiley and Sons, 1974), cited by Conwell, p. 71.

9. Conwell, *op. cit.*, pp. 72–73.

10. *Washington Post*, Aug. 24, 1975, p. A–4.

11. Conwell, *op. cit.*, p. 74, cites evidence that 71 per cent of student nurses felt poorly prepared to deal with death and bereavement.

12. Personal interview.

13. A. L. Strauss and G. G. Glaser. *Anguish: A Case History of a Dying Projectory* (Mill Valley, Calif.: The Sociology Press, 1970).

14. In Stewart, *op. cit.*

15. Stewart, *op. cit.*, p. 69.

16. *Ibid.*

Chapter 4. The Hospice Concept in England

1. This history is summarized in Lamerton, *op. cit.*, and on pages 164 ff of the *October 1976 Report of the Palliative Care Service, Pilot Project January 1975–1977*, Royal Victoria Hospital, McGill University, Montreal, Canada, where the hospice concept is also traced to the concept of medieval French hospitals.

2. *Ibid.*, and "Hospice Britain," in *Senior Citizen News*, May 1976.

3. L. M. Liegner, "St. Christopher's Hospice," *Journal of the American Medical Association*, Dec. 8, 1975.

4. *Ibid.*

5. Joan Kron, "Designing a Better Place to Die," *New York Magazine*, Mar. 1, 1976.

6. *Ibid.*

7. *Ibid.*, p. 46.

8. Thelma Ingles, "St. Christopher's Hospice," *Nursing Outlook*, December 1974.

9. Liegner, *op. cit.*

10. Lamerton, *op. cit.*, p. 85.

11. From a lecture by Dr. Sylvia Lack at a New Haven Hospice consultation.

12. *Ibid.*

13. Lamerton, *op. cit.*, p. 56.

14. *Ibid.*

15. *Ibid.*

16. R. G. Twycross, "Diseases of the Central Nervous System: Relief of Terminal Pain," *British Medical Journal*, Oct. 25, 1975.

17. Lamerton, *op. cit.*, p. 48.

18. *Ibid.*, p. 49.

19. *Ibid.*, pp. 1–7.

20. Twycross, *op. cit.*

21. C. Holden, "Hospices, etc.," *op. cit.*

22. Joan Craven and Florence J. Wald, "Care of the Dying," *Lancet*, October 1971, p. 1822.

23. Lamerton, *op. cit.*, pp. 59–60.

24. From Lamerton, *op. cit.*

25. *Ibid.*

26. *Ibid.*

Chapter 5. The New Haven Hospice: An American Adaptation

1. The New Haven hospice program is designated the Branford Hospice after the suburb where property has been purchased to erect a facility.

2. See "A Prophetic Ministry to the Dying; An Interview with Edward Dobihal," *Christian Century*, Apr. 21, 1976.

3. Kübler-Ross, *On Death and Dying, op. cit.*, pp. 8–9.

4. From a lecture at a New Haven Hospice Consultation.

5. Seymour Sarasen. *The Creation of Settings* (San Francisco: Jossey-Bass, 1972).

6. Joan Kron, "Designing a Better Place to Die," *New York Magazine*, Mar. 1, 1976.

7. *Ibid.* Much of the information about architecture is adapted from this article.

8. See Murray Parkes, *op. cit.*

9. Kron, *op. cit.*

10. *Newsweek*, Jan. 6, 1975.

11. Stewart Alsop. *Stay of Execution* (Philadelphia: Lippincott, 1973).

12. Walter Modell. *Relief of Symptoms* (St. Louis: C. V. Mosby Co., 1961), p. 79.

13. Arthur Lipman, "Drug Therapy in Terminally Ill Patients," *American Journal of Hospital Pharmacists*, 32: 270–276; March 1975.

14. B. M. Mount, I. Ajemian, J. F. Scott, "Use of the Brompton Mixture in Treating the Chronic Pain of Malignant Disease," *Canadian Medical Association Journal,* July 17, 1976, p. 122.

15. Modell, *op. cit.,* p. 63.

16. Mount, *op. cit.*

17. *October 1976 Report, Palliative Care Service, Royal Victoria Hospital, op. cit.,* pp. 168 ff.

18. *Ibid.*

Chapter 6. Challenges and Alternatives

1. See Jim Garner, "Palliative Care: It's the Quality of Life Remaining That Matters," *Canadian Medical Association Journal,* July 17, 1976, pp. 178 ff.

2. From Yeates Conwell, "Toward an Ideal System of Care for the Terminally Ill," *op. cit.,* Chap. I.

3. See definition statement at beginning of this volume.

4. See *October 1976 Report of the Palliative Care Service, Royal Victoria Hospital, op. cit.,* pp. 162–63 and following.

5. *Ibid.,* p. 154.

6. "Calvary Gives Terminal Patients an 'Integrated' Approach to Death," reprinted from a J. B. Barden article in the *New York Times.* Calvary Hospital, 1600 Macombs Road, Bronx, N.Y. 10452.

7. Material from interviews by Conwell, *op. cit.,* Chap. III.

8. From J. J. Walsh. *Mother Alphonse: Rose Hawthorne Lathrop* (New York: Macmillan Co., 1930). Also see T. Maynard. *A Fire Was Lighted* (Milwaukee: Bruce, 1948), and M. Vance. *On Wings of Fire* (New York: Dutton, 1950).

9. Jerome Singer, "Fantasy, the Foundation of Serenity," *Psychology Today,* July, 1975, pp. 32 ff.

10. Marya Mannes. *Last Rights* (New York: Wm. Morrow, 1974), Chap. XV.

11. Note, *October 1976 Report of the Palliative Care Service, op. cit.,* p. 26, discussion of a music therapist at Royal Victoria Hospital.

12. *Ibid.*, p. 2.

13. International Seminar on Terminal Care, Nov. 3–5, 1976

14. *Oct. 1976 Report of the Palliative Care Service, op. cit.*, p. 16.

15. *Ibid.*, p. 28.

16. *Ibid.*, p. 39.

17. Krant, *op. cit.*, pp. 143–44.

18. In Holden, C., *op. cit.* p. 391.

Chapter 7. The Hospice Concept as Program

1. "Hospice, A Pilot Project," St. Luke's Hospital Center, November 1975.

2. *Ibid.*, pp. 2–3.

3. *October 1976 Report of the Palliative Care Service, Royal Victoria Hospital, op. cit.*, p. 103.

4. *Ibid.*, p. 111.

5. "Hospice, A Pilot Project," St Luke's, *op. cit.*

6. *Ibid.*, p. 9.

7. *October 1976 Report, Royal Victoria, op. cit.*, p. 76.

8. *Ibid.*, p. 73.

9. *Ibid.*, p. 118.

10. *Ibid.*, p. 197.

11. *Ibid.*, pp. 250–255.

12. *Ibid.*, pp. 258 ff.

13. Lamerton, "Care of the Dying," *op. cit.*, pp. 54–56.

14. Parker Rossman, "So You Are Going to the Trappists, An Interview with Henri Nouwen," *Christian Century*, Oct. 2, 1974.

15. *Archives of the Foundation of Thanatology, 1975*, contains summaries of a number of studies of the work of volunteers with the terminally ill.

16. Louise Jaffe, University of Pittsburgh Department of Social Work.

17. See *October 1976 Report, Royal Victoria, op. cit.*, pp. 313–315.

18. B. D. Colen, "Ten Bad Days Among the Dying," *Washington Post*, Oct. 31, 1976.

19. *October 1976 Report, Royal Victoria, op. cit.*, pp. 478 ff.

20. *Ibid.*, p. 137.

21. *Ibid.*

Chapter 8. Advice to Other Communities

1. C. Holden, *op. cit.*, p. 391.
2. Mannes, *op. cit.*
3. John DeBoer. *Let's Plan* (Philadelphia: Pilgrim Press, 1970).
4. See "Hospice: A Pilot Project," St. Luke's Hospital Center, Amsterdam Ave. at 114th Street, New York, N.Y. 10025; and "To Honor All of Life: A National Demonstration Center to Protect the Rights of the Terminally Ill" (the case for the support of Hospice, Inc., 765 Prospect St., New Haven, CT 06511), and documentation from the Palliative Care Unit of Royal Victoria Hospital, McGill University, Montreal, Quebec, Canada.

Chapter 9. Some Financial Aspects

1. H. Jack Geiger, from book review of *Blue Cross: What Went Wrong?* by Sylvia A. Law and the Health Law Project at the University of Pennsylvania, *New York Times Book Review*, June 23, 1974.
2. See Seymour Harris. *The Economics of Modern Medicine* (New York: Macmillan Co., 1964).
3. Geiger, *op. cit.*
4. Harry Schwartz, "On Medical Progress," *New York Times*, Apr. 13, 1976, p. 33.
5. Geiger, *op. cit.*
6. From a lecture by Dr. Colin Murray Parkes, see Parkes, *op. cit.*
7. Garner, *op. cit.*
8. See *1976 Report, Palliative Care Unit, Royal Victoria Hospital, op. cit.* p. 195, p. 309.
9. 1976 Annual Report, New Haven Hospice.
10. Connecticut House Bill No. 7467, Public Act No. 75–623, January 1975.
11. Yeates Conwell, *op. cit.*, pp. 7 ff.

Chapter 10. Caring for the Dying at Home

1. R. C. Fox, and J. P. Swazey. *The Courage to Fail: A Social View of Organ Transplantation and Dialysis* (Chicago: University of Chicago Press, 1974), p. 336.
2. Fred J. Cook. *Julia's Story* (New York: Holt, Rinehart & Winston, 1976).

3. Jane Brody, reviewing *Julia's Story*, *New York Times Book Review*, June 29, 1976, p. 29.

4. Twycross, *op. cit.*

5. David Duncombe, "Finishing Unfinished Business," an address to a hospice group in New York State, Nov. 12, 1976.

6. This section quoted from "To Honor All of Life," *op. cit.*, pp. 23–24.

7. Stanley Lesse, M.D., "The Preventive Psychiatry of the Future," *The Futurist*, October 1976, pp. 228 ff.

8. Rabitha M. Powledge, "Death as an Acceptable Subject," *New York Times*, July 25, 1976.

9. "To Honor All of Life," *op. cit.*

10. *Ibid.*

Appendix I: Materials Used in Orienting Volunteers

The Palliative Care Service at Royal Victoria Hospital in Montreal, Canada, recommends:

For Reading: Kübler-Ross, E. *On Death and Dying*. New York: Macmillan, 1973.

Hinton, J. *Dying*. London: Penguin, 1967.

Parkes, C. M. *Bereavement*. New York: International Universities Press, 1972.

16-mm. films: "To Die Today," Dr. Elisabeth Kübler-Ross, on fear of death, a patient interview, 55 minutes, Filmmakers Library, U.S.A.

"Death," Calvary Hospital, New York City, 40 minutes. Filmmakers Library, U.S.A.

"The Gift," program from "The Waltons" where a friend is dying of leukemia, 55 minutes, Warner Brothers.

Audiotape: "Death, Grief, and Bereavement," from the Center for Death Education and Research, University of Minnesota. Also bibliographies from this source.

Videotapes: The Palliative Care Service at Royal Victoria Hospital has for its own use taped "Thoughts on Dying," an interview with Dr. Balfour Mount; "Bereavement," with Dr. Colin Murray Parkes; "Interview with Miss C.," the spiritual and philosophical views of a dying patient; "Participant Observation," with Dr. Mount, Dr. I. Ajemian, and the director of research of New Haven Hospice, Robert Buckingham.

Color film strip: "Perspectives on Dying," from Concept Media with six cassettes: "American Attitudes Toward Death and Dying," "Psychological Reactions of Dying Persons," "Hazards and Challenges in Providing Care," and so on.

Hospice

AN OFFICIAL DEFINITION

Hospice: a program which provides palliative and supportive care for terminally-ill patients and their families, either directly or on a *consulting* basis with the patient's physician or another community agency such as a Visiting Nurse Association. Originally a medieval name for a way station for pilgrims and travelers where they could be replenished, refreshed, and cared for; used here for an organized program of care for people going through life's last station. The whole family is considered the unit of care, and care extends through the mourning process. Emphasis is placed on symptom control and preparation for and support before and after death, full-scope health services being provided for by an organized interdisciplinary team available on a twenty-four-hour-a-day, seven-day-a-week basis. Hospices originated in England (where there are about 25) and are now appearing in the United States. As one example of their human- and cost-saving effects, 61 per cent of one hospice's patients died at home (compared with the 2 per cent of all American deaths which occur at home.)

HOSPICE GOALS

1. Keep patient at home as long as possible.
2. Supplement, not duplicate, existing services.
3. Educate: health professionals, lay people.
4. Support family as unit of care.
5. Help patient to live as fully as possible.
6. Keep costs down.

From *A Discursive Dictionary of Health Care*, prepared by the Staff for the use of the Subcommittee on Health and the Environment of the Committee on Interstate and Foreign Commerce, U.S. House of Representatives, February, 1976.